KILLER

BOOBS

A BREAST CANCER MEMOIR

Amy Valentine

Personville Press
HOUSTON, TEXAS

Personville Press
6121 Winsome Lane #56C
Houston, TX 77057
USA
www.personvillepress.com

You can follow the author's blog at www.amyshealth.com . To contact the author, write amyvalentine@gmail.com

This is the first volume of a series. The next volume (titled *Cleavage to Die For*) will be out in 2014.

Book Layout ©2013 BookDesignTemplates.com
Cover Design by Allison Mabry.
Editorial assistance by Robert Nagle.
Printed by CreateSpace.
An ebook version of this title is available. Check the author's site for details.

Quantity sales. Special discounts are available on quantity purchases by corporations, associations, and others. For details, contact the author or the publisher.

Killer Boobs/ Amy Valentine. -- 1st print ed.
ISBN978-1493523306
I. Personal Memoir II. Breast Cancer

Perhaps none of us knows the extent of human kindness unless faced with a devastating medical challenge. And few of us fathom the depth of our internal strength and resiliency until tested.

"Yes, they're fake. My real ones tried to kill me."

—T SHIRT SLOGAN

Contents

Day 1 to 15   **1**

Day 22 to 122   **23**

Day 115 to 153   **69**

Day 154 to 250   **89**

About the Author   **129**

Day 1 to 15

On March 27, 2009, I was a 42 year old, stay-at-home wife and mother to a three and five year old. I was also about to be diagnosed with Stage 3, triple-positive, bilateral breast cancer, with five tumors across both breasts. My world fell apart, then I began to put one foot in front of the other, because in the crazy cancer world I was about to enter, that was the only way to reach the other side.

Day 1

I've never been "felt up" so much as the week following my Stage III breast cancer diagnosis. "Where are you now?" my husband's slightly frantic voice on the cell phone asked.

"Driving to the surgeon's for a biopsy."

"Okay..." he stalled as he processed this new bit of information. The last we had spoken, he was in the airport in another state awaiting his return flight home to Austin, Texas from a business trip. I was at the mammography center waiting to hear the radiologist's report on my diagnostic mammogram and ultrasound.

"The radiologists wanted a biopsy and Dr. M had to order it, so she told me she'd make some phone calls and get me in right away. She found a surgeon that can see me today, so that's where I'm going," I rattled off.

"Got to go, honey, I have another call," I told him, my just-get-it-done mode kicking in as I tried to manage my emotions, juggle the cell phone calls, and drive. No wonder there are so many accidents while people are talking on their phones! How many of them are wondering if they have cancer? I was finding it hard to breathe, let alone drive and talk on the phone at the same time. Pushing that random thought away, I answered my incoming call.

My good friend Di was on the line; "What's going on Amy? Your phone message sounded urgent."

"I showed my lump to Dr. M, who referred me to the women's center for a diagnostic mammogram and ultrasound. The radiologist recommended biopsies on both sides. Dr. M got me in with a surgeon, so I'm driving there." I blurted out my story as I switched lanes and almost dropped the phone in my lap.

"When is the appointment? Who's going with you?"

"Whenever I get there. The surgeon said he would wait for me to get Daniel and Sara's childcare taken care of. I'm going by myself since Greg's still out of town."

"I'll come with you. Where is it?"

Thank God for Di, because a breast biopsy is best experienced with a good friend or relative. If nothing else, it gives the patient a reason to act bravely, and a shoulder to cry on when the news isn't the best.

As a stay-at-home mother of two young children, 4 year old Daniel and 6 year old Sara, who had just begun a new children's cooking business, I didn't have time for this healthcare complication. My husband Greg and I had been married seven years.

I still didn't think there would be anything wrong with my breast. My mother had lumpy breasts like mine and had undergone numerous biopsies over the years and none of them had turned out to be anything requiring further treatment. There was no history of cancer in our family, and I was only 42. I just needed to take care of this. Now!

Twenty minutes later Di joined me in the exam room where the nurse had left me a garment resembling a poncho. Instead of a traditional hospital gown, this was a square piece of cloth with a hole cut out where the patient's head would go. My ob/gyn already had me put on a similarly bizarre looking garment earlier that day, so I recognized what to do with it. Di, however, had never seen it and was amazed when I stripped and popped the poncho over my head.

"What the hell is that?"

"Breast poncho," I replied not missing a beat, amused at her expression.

"I kinda think it's sexy. It's really short and just covers your breasts," Di said.

"Yeah, sexy. That's exactly what I'm thinking right now," I deadpanned, happy that my sense of humor was still with me during this panicky emotional state.

Just then, the door opened and the surgeon and his nurse entered. After a few pleasantries, he began discussing my lump. It's a funny word, pleasantries, when the small talk was anything but pleasant due to the fact that the words "biopsy," "suspicious lump" and "cancer" were hanging in the air. The doctor kept leading the conversation to treatment for cancer, and I kept leading it away.

"What happens if we do the biopsy and it's normal?" I asked.

"We still need to take it out. No 42 year old woman should have a hard lump in her breast."

I laid back on the exam table with my arms above my head, purposefully looking away from the surgeon on my right side where the offending lump had invaded my breast.

"First, let me show you the biopsy tool so you'll know what to expect," Dr. W said, holding up what looked like an ear piercing machine from a store in the mall. "I'm going to numb your skin and use the ultrasound machine to find the lump. Then I'll push against your breast with this machine until I get it in place. After that, I pull this trigger and it will make a loud sound when the needle shoots out to take the core biopsy. Like this."

Dr. W pulled the trigger and the machine made a loud mechanical similar to that of one of my four-year-old son's toys.

"You're kidding me, right?" I said.

I couldn't believe this archaic instrument was really how surgeons' biopsy breasts in the 21st century. I momentarily considered getting dressed and finding a surgeon who had less medieval equipment. Or, offering to give the doctor $100 to buy one of the newfangled biopsy instruments that I was sure were available in 2009. But I remembered that my ob/gyn (whom I've known for 20 years, and trusted completely) sent me to this surgeon. I said nothing and laid back down on the exam table.

Dr. W proceeded to use the ultrasound machine and goopy gel to find the lump, and then leaned on me in a way that would have been uncomfortable except for the fact that I just wanted to get this over with as quickly as possible. I'm not sure there was anything any medical professional could have done to me that day that would have caused me to complain, no matter how painful or uncomfortable or awkward.

I mentally counted up the number of medical professionals who had felt my breasts that day. First was my ob/gyn, then the mammogram tech, the ultrasound tech, and now the surgeon. If I were in high school, this would be a very popular day!

At one point, the doctor said to my friend Di, who had remained in the room: "Don't look over here at all this blood. It looks like Bagdad but it's not that bad, really. The ultrasound gel makes the blood runny and it looks much worse than it is."

Fortunately, Di was a safari hunter and had seen much worse than blood. For some reason as she explained to the doctor that she was not frightened by the sight of blood, I thought of my grandfather. He was a kind, gentle soul who showed good will towards every person he encountered and said he had never met a stranger. One Thanksgiving in my teens I cut my finger while deboning the holiday turkey. My grandfather and I debated going to the emergency room because the cut was so deep. After seeing my finger, my grandfather had to sit down. I asked him if he grew faint at the sight of blood.

"No," he said. "Only at the sight of your blood." Sweet, sweet man.

After the assault on my lumpy breast was complete and I was bandaged and dressed, the surgeon explained that he'd like to order an MRI for my second breast, because it had some tiny abnormalities that couldn't be seen clearly in the mammogram or ultrasound. He then explained that he would have the pathology report from the biopsy the next day.

Since all this talk was quite somber, I cheerfully replied, "I'll just assume my lump is benign then, until I hear from you."

The surgeon paused for a fraction of a second as he looked for the best phrasing to prepare me for what was to come, because he knew the truth from my exams. They all knew. The mammogram tech, the ultrasound tech, the radiologist, the surgeon.

"Well...your mammogram was troubling, your ultrasound was troubling, and I didn't like the look of the cells I pulled from your body."

That's when my world fell apart.

Day 2

My husband Greg, just home from his business trip, stayed home with me the next day to await the pathology results. I thought the surgeon had said he would have results by noon, so when 12 o'clock came and went, I called his office. A nurse told me Dr. W wouldn't have an official pathology report until Monday, giving me a reprieve of sorts over the weekend.

So, when the phone rang and Dr. W began, "Amy, I have your pathology report and it's bad news..." I stopped him by saying, "but, your nurse told me you wouldn't have the official pathology report until noon. You can't be giving me bad news!"

As if I could negate the words I had just heard him tell me.

"I don't have an official pathology report," Dr. W said, "but I was so concerned about your report that I walked over to the pathologist's office and waited while he looked at your cells under the microscope."

Wow.

Then he asked something I found rather funny, even in my shell-shocked state.

"Do you have an oncologist?"

"Excuse me?"

"Do you have an oncologist, or would you like me to call and get you an appointment? If you would like me to call, you would probably be able to arrange the appointment more quickly," my helpful surgeon said.

"Ok."

As if I had an entourage of medical specialists waiting for the moment in time that I would need them. A gastroenterologist for the colonoscopy that would be in my future and a cardiologist for the unknown heart trouble in my 70s and a rheumatologist for the arthritis that would cripple me forty years in the future.

My next phone call was to my ob/gyn. Since the surgeon had discussed my case with her prior to calling me, she was already aware of the results. When I gave my name to the receptionist, my physician immediately picked up the phone, as if she had been waiting for my call.

"I'm so sorry, Amy," were her words and I thought how hard it must be for doctors to know their patients might die. And to have conversations with them about their disease.

I told her my husband had asked me to get a prescription for Valium and my ob/gyn asked, "For you or for him?" Hard to say at that point.

She called in 30 Xanax.

Two years later I still had the same bottle of calming drugs, and realized I had only taken three quarters of the bottle, most of them consumed that first weekend after diagnosis. Strange how you can rally when you need to. Would I have risen to the challenge ahead of me if I had known what was in store? Ignorance is bliss in some cases.

My surgeon had ordered a chest MRI to see about the mysterious calcifications in my left breast, since no lump or bump was big enough for him to biopsy.

"I'm worried about claustrophobia in the MRI machine," I told Greg.

"Why don't you take an extra Xanax pill before the exam?" he suggested, so I did.

I fell asleep in the machine, which seemed to be a first for the MRI techs.

As we left the painless MRI procedure, I realized how minimally invasive it had been and how difficult the road ahead of me was going to be. I thought of how scary it would be for our 4 and 6 year old children to go through an MRI, let alone any other as-yet-unrevealed procedure ahead of me, and I felt a surge of gratitude. Somehow this marked a turning point for me as I contemplated the challenges ahead. I could do this. Better me than my children.

"I'm so glad this is me and not Sara or Daniel," I whispered to Greg as we walked hand-in-hand back to our car, still groggy from the drugs and my nap.

"I wish it were me," he said, giving my hand a squeeze. For my stoic computer engineer husband, that was an emotional outburst.

Later, this same quiet husband would set up my own website enabling me to blog about my cancer experience, knowing that the writer in me needed a cathartic outlet.

"I want nothing to do with a cancer blog," I complained to my best friend Julie. "I don't want to talk about my cancer. I don't want to think about my cancer." As if I could do anything *except* think about cancer.

I didn't even like to touch my breasts in the shower, knowing they were trying to kill me.

"This is your quiet computer geek husband's way of showing support," Julie chastised me when I complained about the expectation that I blog. "You go write one paragraph on that website, and you thank Greg for setting it up for you. One paragraph. Go do it," she commanded.

I respond well to direct orders.

I blogged. And found it cathartic and encouraging and meaningful. In writing about my experiences I discovered I could focus on the surreal, bizarre and unbelievable, because everything has a touch of humor in it, given the right viewpoint, even cancer.

I mean, given such good comedic material as the cancer world, how could I not find it funny?

Day 8

"You seem really healthy," my oncologist Dr. K said after his initial physical exam. In fact he would make that comment after each and every visit, and I saw him a lot that first month.

"Yes, except for this cancer you say I have," I would reply in a sarcastic tone. To his inquiry about how I had been feeling over the past few months, I said, "hmmm, am I tired? I have a 4-year-old and a 6-year-old and I'm 42. Yes, I'm tired but I blame it more on the children than the cancer."

"Do you have a family history of cancer?"

"No, unless you count my grandfather who died of colon cancer."

"Tell me more about him," Dr. K said, perking up visibly at some family history of cancer, because he liked to know the answers to puzzles. Why he became an oncologist I'll never know. It must be a frustrating career choice because there never seems to be a clear answer in this field. Who gets cancer? Why does someone get cancer? Why do some people die and others survive? The majority of patients don't have a family history. Why not be a surgeon? Cut out the problem and send the patient on his way. An oncologist deals with the unexplainable every day.

"Well, my Dad's father died of colon cancer," I answered, waiting a beat for the kicker. "When he was 97." I felt a little bit bad for Dr. K and his obvious disappointment in my true lack of family cancer history.

Oh, bad Amy. Taking out frustrations by teasing the nice oncologist!

"At that age, we'll all get something…" Dr. K says, deflated by my grandfather's advanced age when developing cancer. "I'm not going to write down your 97-year-old grandfather as a family history of cancer."

I fully expected to open my veins for chemo that first oncology visit, wanting to get rid of this disease. Dr. K slowed me down by explaining they needed to know more about the type of breast cancer and all of its receptors, and how far it had spread so they would know what type of treatment I would need. They wanted to check for the BRAC gene to see if there were a genetic predisposition to breast, colon and ovarian cancer. We discussed lumpectomy and radiation followed by some Tamoxifen pills. This all seemed a bit minor to me. I expected months of chemo and asked about a mastectomy at that point, knowing my lumpy breasts would continue to haunt me each month if I kept them. Plus, they wanted to kill me. Why did I want to keep them around?

I told the doctor, "I want to be aggressive. Take off my arms and legs but give me 20 years. I have small children at home."

Whenever I would invoke the "20 years" timeframe in my negotiations with God, I would realize at some point that I would only be 62 at that time, young to die by anyone's estimate.

That was the nature of my bartering prayers during the early days of my diagnosis. Isn't that one of the seven stages of grief? Bargaining? I began most conversations with God, "take whatever you want, do whatever must be done to me, but give me 20 years to mother my children."

"How exactly will this cancer kill me if we leave it alone? Isn't that an option?" I asked my doctor at my initial visit. "I feel fine now and I know you are going to make me feel awful."

"Well, if left untreated, the cancer cells will continue to grow and spread, looking for soft tissue like the liver, lungs or bones to attack. Then, you will have trouble with those organs. That will bring a great deal of discomfort and ultimately cause the body to stop functioning the way it should."

"Okay, then." I said, cowed by his gruesome explanation. "Let's get rid of it." As if there had ever been a doubt that I was going to fight the disease.

A funny letter came from The Breast Center, about two weeks after my diagnosis, when I was in the midst of staging and treatment and surgery appointments. It said I had an abnormality on my mammogram and needed to see my physician. Greg commented, "Get right on that."

On April 1st, five days after my diagnosis, no one called to tell me this nightmare was all a bad April Fool's joke.

As part of the staging to see how far the cancer had already spread inside me, my oncologist ordered a chest and abdomen CT and a nuclear bone scan. The three main areas breast cancer likes to spread to are the liver, lungs and bones.

At my chest and abdomen CT scans, the tech told me she'd been seeing lots more young folks (both women and men) with breast cancer, which was really unusual. I had to drink some gross liquid but the worse part of the procedure was right before the CT exam. The tech has me eat a few spoonfuls of a paste to highlight my esophagus. She compared it to flan.

I hate flan. This was my own particular hell and at that moment I had an internal conversation with God.

"Really, God? First cancer, now flan-like paste? I'm starting to lose my sense of humor."

But, I wasn't going to let a little flan barium paste hold me down. So I mushed it around my mouth and somehow swallowed the icky substance.

Then I had the nuclear dye injected in my veins for the bone scan to see if the cancer had already invaded my bone marrow. That was an easy test, but scary in the thought that the radiologists might be seeing little blips that signaled metastasized cancer.

After the morning barrage of tests I collapsed, absolutely exhausted. I found it hard to think. But even harder to think about anything except cancer.

I complained about the CT scan and the barium flan-like paste, but there was a bright moment in the procedure. While I was hooked up to an IV in the CT machine, the techs injected a contrast dye into the IV that felt hot as it ran through my body. The tech told me I would feel like I was peeing myself, but I wouldn't really.

The CT machine has a male voice programmed into it with a British accent,

"Hold your breath now please."

"You may resume breathing."

I found that oddly surreal and amusing. Where did this British bloke come from? Why does a breast cancer patient in Austin get the British voice-over telling her to "resume breathing?"

The tech injected the dye and the CT started scanning. I felt the hot liquid coursing through my body and yes, as it settled in my nether regions, it did feel like I was peeing myself.

But, the warm tingling sensation wasn't all unpleasant. (Cue sexy music here.)

I involuntarily began laughing. "My husband is right outside in the waiting room if you'd be so kind as to bring him in. This is kinda putting me in the mood."

As the tech was taking me off the machine, she commented, "Oh yes, you're premenopausal. I guess that warm contrast dye had a different effect on you than on older folks." Bow chick a bow wow…

Of course, my normal life of being a mom to two young children continued despite my cancer diagnosis.

Two days later, I had to take Daniel to the pediatrician for a small rash that hadn't cleared up.

"So, I've been diagnosed with breast cancer," I said to our pediatrician.

"I'm so sorry to hear that, you see to be taking this rather calmly."

"Well, that's probably the drugs," I deadpanned. "But, I'm not going anywhere. I have a 4 and 6 year old."

"Of course you'll be fine. Did I ever wonder where Sara got her spunky nature?"

That became my mantra: I'm spunky and I'll be fine. I'm spunky and I'll be fine. I'm spunky and I'll be fine....

The only true risk factor I had was having my first child after the age of 30. I thought of how many I knew who'd also waited until after their twenties to conceive. What if I had married my college sweetheart and had children early? Would that have prevented my cancer?

I asked my husband if he thought I'd ever know what caused my cancer.

"When I die, do you think I get to ask God why I got cancer?"

"Do you really think that's what you're going to ask God when you die?" he queried.

"No," I said, thinking about it, "I want to know what happened to Jon Benet Ramsey."

Day 10

When walking to school this morning, six-year-old Sara took my hand and said she wished it were she who had cancer. I squeezed her little hand and said, "No honey, it's better that it happened to me. I'm older than you." Sara answered, "Yes, that's it. I'm younger and have fewer memories, so if I die, I'd have fewer things to miss about life." I couldn't speak. Damn this cancer.

"Stop trolling the Internet," Greg commanded, because that's what I did, curious about this mysterious disease that was trying to kill me. When you've been recently diagnosed with cancer, nothing you find online is good. No news was encouraging. I found a website where women could calculate their risk of developing breast cancer. When I entered my stats, pretending I had taken this quiz in February instead of in March, I found out I had less than a one percent chance of getting breast cancer. Great. I'm such a rebel.

My mother, who has always had lumpy breasts, like mine, goes for a check up and reminds me that having a family member with breast cancer has now increased her chances of contracting the disease. We both laugh at the ridiculousness of the situation.

Several women friends of mine asked me about the lump in my breast, curious what a cancerous lump felt like.

When my friend Di was over visiting, she told me her breasts weren't lumpy. They were always soft. So, we proceeded to feel each other's breasts, curious as to the different types of breast consistency.

Greg looked up and said, "Can I videotape this?"

Along with avoiding my temptation to troll the Internet for statistics on breast cancer divorce rates, five year survival rates, and possible causes of cancer, I had also limited my conversations with other breast cancer patients/friends/relatives.

The situation reminded me of my single, dating years. Someone would set me up on a date with a man and the only thing we had in common was that we were both single.

Folks kept referring me to their friends/relatives etc. who also have had breast cancer. But, unless they have had my version of triple positive cancer, at my stage IIIA, managing two young children at home, their experience didn't have much to do with me.

Plus, I got cancer-envy. I heard stories of people who had "better" cancers than me. The kind that don't really grow fast. The kind that were still *in situ* inside the duct while mine started acting up and moved into the regular breast tissue.

"I'm sure all those pancreatic cancer patients would be happy to trade you for your breast cancer," my down-to-earth friend Julie reminded me, refusing to allow me to feel sorry for myself.

Day 15

The plastic surgeon's office was fancy, with a waterfall art sculpture on the entry wall and a beautiful receptionist greeting patients. Was she a subtle advertisement for the doctor's services?

"Look, instead of the thick cotton exam gowns, I have this plush bathrobe!" I said excitedly to Greg and Di, who had accompanied me.

I developed an immediate crush on my plastic surgeon, based mainly on the fact that he was a physician who didn't seem very interested in my cancer. He was more interested in the reconstruction process. It was a breath of fresh air.

I was seated on the exam table at table height while Dr. H was on a rolling stool, about level with my chest. He pulled himself up to the exam table, in a rather suggestive position between my legs with his face at my breast level. Then, he slowly pulled the plush bathrobe off my shoulders. Dr. H gently poked and pinched me. Is there a wonder I developed a crush?

"You have good material to work with," he complimented my diseased breasts.

Greg commented under his breath, "I've always said you had good breasts" and Di gave him a playful slap. If we weren't dealing with cancer, this whole scene would be hilarious!

I had always liked my breasts. Now, however, now they were trying to kill me. Damned ungrateful boobs. After all the kindnesses I've shown them – pretty bras, trips to the beach, nursing babies. Sigh.

Then, Dr. H explained the bizarre reconstruction process. After the initial mastectomy surgery, in which my general surgeon and plastic surgeon would operate, and a two to three week recovery period, I would see Dr. H every three weeks and he would fill my expanders with fluid to stretch the skin.

"Once you reach the size we want," he continued, "we stop filling the expanders and wait three months for scar tissue to form around the expander balloon."

This would all occur during my four to six months of chemo, if that became part of my treatment plan. At this point, we didn't know the extent of my disease or what that treatment would consist of. Dr. H told me the expander is a hard, big balloon so I would seem really big for several months.

"Step two would be an outpatient procedure under general anesthesia," he continued. "At that time, the expanders are removed, and replaced with silicone gel implants."

Remember, I would have no nipples at this point. Although, if I would be in the midst of chemotherapy, I think nipples would be at the bottom of my list of concerns! I laughed about having a nose job too since my insurance would already be paying for the surgical suite and the anesthesia. The nurse said tons of folks do cosmetic procedures at this point. Hmmm, tummy tuck? Eyelid lift? Nose job? Endless possibilities...

Step three would be when Dr. H would create nipples by bunching the skin into a nipple-shaped fold. Someone in the plastic surgeon's office would then tattoo the appropriate color onto the nipple.

After we all absorbed the information, Di said to the nurse, "Does this visit come with a glass of wine?"

"I would have already drunk it," she replied. "I'm having a tough week painting and moving into my new house."

"Trade you," I immediately said. My cancer was making me snarky.

Day 22 to 112

"**H**ave you come to say goodbye to the girls?" I asked my ob/gyn as she came into the pre-op waiting room before my double mastectomy surgery.

"No, I'm here to say goodbye to the cancer."

Good one, I thought. Being naturally witty (or perhaps just a smart ass), I'm always impressed when someone one-ups my attempt at humor.

Years ago, a friend of mine had her first child by planned cesarean section. When I went to visit her in the hospital, she said the experience was a bit like taking a trip. She had to pack a bag and leave the house before dawn. Checking in at the hospital was almost like checking in at the airport with all the questions and kiosks and clerks.

My mastectomy experience should have been like that. We packed a bag and got to the hospital before dawn. We had to check in at several desks and visit several different clerks, the most important one being the "insurance counselor."

The surgery from the hospital's point of view would cost approximately $70,000, not including those extras like the surgeon, anesthesiologist and any other medical necessities. With my nice insurance, the hospital would receive approximately $7,000. I would be responsible for my 10 percent or $700. Would that be cash, check or charge?

Just for kicks, I asked the financial counselor what would happen if I hadn't had insurance. Would I be asked to pay the $7,000?

He replied, "no, you would be billed the full $70K."

"What?" I was confused. "But you accepted $7,000 for the surgery from the insurance company. Why wouldn't you accept that same amount from another person if they didn't have insurance coverage bringing their portion down?"

The answer was that if the hospital routinely accepted $7,000, then the insurance companies would begin discounting their allowable rate and wouldn't pay $7,000. And who are these folks who think we don't need healthcare reform in this country?

By the way, while I don't recommend having a double mastectomy, if you do, bring your own calming drugs to the morning of surgery. Anticipating a few hours of wait time before surgery, I called the pre-op nurse a few days earlier.

"Should I bring my Xanax to surgery the day of my procedure?"

The nurse replied, "We have the good stuff here for you, so don't worry about bringing your own. The doctor wants to talk to you before the surgery so he would prefer you aren't drugged up before you get here."

Bad advice!

No one gave me drugs until about two minutes before my actual surgery. Personally, if you have to go in the hospital for a double mastectomy, I suggest you take it upon yourself to take some drugs beforehand. I would've been much happier with a Xanax or two in me.

One of the most painful procedures of my entire cancer ordeal was the dye procedure to find the sentinel lymph nodes, done a few hours before my mastectomy.

The radiologist injected dye into the nipples and then waited for it to travel to the lymph nodes in order for the surgeon to be able to detect the ones possibly affected by cancer. A friend of mine from the children's preschool was the radiologist on duty that day and she had helpfully requested to do the procedure herself, which gave me some clout in the radiology suite.

Not that it bought me anything, but the techs all jumped around and treated me as if I were a VIP. Maybe they do that to all breast cancer patients. After all, it is true that most people are nice to cancer patients, especially bald ones who are obviously going through chemo.

"This might sting some," Dr. Liz said, "so we inject a numbing solution first, then the dye." Aichee-Momma! Yes, it stung. And continued to burn as it moved around my breast.

Then, after waiting an agonizing 20 minutes for the dye to do its job, the techs put metal plates on top of my nipples to mask the injection site, and took x-rays to find the sentinel lymph nodes. All in all, it was not a fun experience. And, why didn't I get any Xanax before this hell?

Later, I tried to commiserate with a fellow breast cancer patient in the chemo infusion room, assuming all women had to endure this same nipple burning hell. She acted shocked, and said her surgeon had performed the sentinel dye procedure after she was already under anesthesia. Great, I had the sadistic surgeon. And he seemed so nice.

"Why didn't my cruel surgeon do the painful sentinel dye procedure after I was knocked out for the surgery?" I complained to my radiologist friend when next I saw her at a preschool function.

Her comment was, "It's standard procedure to perform the sentinel dye before surgery, so I don't know what the other breast cancer patient was talking about. It takes an hour or so to complete, and if you wait to do that under general anesthesia, that just prolongs the time spent under. And no one wants to spend more time under general anesthesia than necessary."

In my mind, I disagreed. I could think of whole days that I wouldn't have minded spending under general anesthesia.

Months later at a mutual friend's child's birthday party, I chatted with this same radiologist. She told me she had discovered how to make the sentinel dye procedure less painful. Instead of injecting the numbing solution before the dye injection, she combined the two in one injection and that seemed to make it more tolerable for the patients.

Couldn't someone before me have complained about the painful procedure so Dr. Liz could have discovered this less-painful version *before* I went in? Sigh.

On the morning of my mastectomy, the doctors finally showed up for my procedure, and the anesthesiologist gave me the happy drugs. They wheeled me into the operating room and had me climb onto the skinny, skinny operating table. I had no idea how skinny the tables were. I was chatting and chatting and I saw someone give the anesthesiologist a hand sign. Apparently, it was "shut her up, already" because a few seconds later, lights out.

The operating room nurse called Greg on his cell phone every hour during the surgery to update him on my progress. Greg put those updates on my cancer blog. A friend of mine traveling to New York City for work said he read the updates on his cell phone throughout the day. He actually stepped into St. Patrick's Cathedral to light a candle on my behalf while I was on the surgical table. Okay, maybe the blog was a good idea.

It was a wild goose chase for my friends and family trying to find me after my surgery, as I was scheduled to be in three different rooms before I wound up in the right one.

"I'm sick of feeling sick," I complained to my husband, who had not left my side in the hospital room since I was taken to the room after surgery and recovery.

Greg slept next to me and ate food friends brought him, along with any food left over on my hospital tray that my nausea had prevented me from eating.

"I can't breathe," I cried to my sleeping husband and insisted that he move me into a more vertical position. I remained nauseous for several days. My left arm tingled. I had moments of anxiety and dizziness when I believed I couldn't breathe and had to be moved into a vertical position to catch my breath even though that increased my nausea.

After two days, I turned a corner ... and got the horrible news that the cancer had spread to lymph nodes on both sides of my body.

"Greg, I'm about to lose my sense of humor about this whole cancer thing," I said, trying to be funny. Neither of us laughed.

Day 27

"Having a double mastectomy is like being a T-Rex dinosaur with these little useless arms you can only wave around at chest height," I said, trying desperately to lift my arms even to shoulder height.

I guess people warned me, but a double mastectomy with reconstruction is a major operation. The anesthesia alone required for a six hour surgery is pretty intense. Maybe it was better I didn't know the full extent of what I was getting myself into, because I never had a second's doubt that I was taking the best possible step in eliminating all sources of problems for the future.

My docs thought I might be a bit too aggressive with going straight to the double mastectomy but after all was said and done, it was definitely a good move.

I woke up from surgery with four drains coming out of my underarms. Blood-tinged ooze had to be drained from them and the liquid measured. Fortunately, my nurse friend Anne came over to help my mom strip and empty my surgical drains and change the dressings.

"I don't see any stitches," I said to Anne.

"Super glue is holding you together," she said, helping me into a shallow warm bath.

"All I want to do is sleep, "I said. But we had a visit to my oncologist to discuss my treatment plan in view of the results of my double mastectomy.

After the exhausting start to the day, my entourage and I went to the oncologist's office to learn about my future. My mom, my brother, Di, and I crowded into a room to hear my oncologist say that he didn't like my cancer.

"I don't like it much either," I commented, always ready with a fast quip to keep myself from crying.

My doc staged me a 3A.

"Big numbers aren't good in the cancer world, right?"

"Yes, it's better to be a Stage 1 than a Stage 2," he replied.

"I don't have an official pathology report yet," my oncologist continued. (What's the story with the late pathology reports? This was getting to be my normal.)

"But I chatted on the phone with the pathologist. On your right side, you had a tumor, which is invasive ductal carcinoma and the cancer had moved into 2 of the 4 lymph nodes. The doctors got it all and were pretty much expecting all of that."

But my left side threw everyone for a loop. I had lots of tiny precancerous *in situ* ductal blobs and two 3 mm invasive ductal carcinoma, but the cancer had also moved into my lymph nodes on that side — 3 of the 4, which was more than on the right side.

"So, both breasts spontaneously decided to go cancerous?" I asked Dr. K.

"Yes, this is normally what we see in someone who tests positive for the BRAC gene defect, which you did not. Blah blah blah."

The doctor didn't actually say "blah blah blah," but at some point, I stopped hearing any more words.

Fortunately, I had brought my posse of friends and family, and Greg called in on his cell phone since he was on a business trip. They listened to the rest of the conversation.

1. It was a good thing we did a double mastectomy because of the extent of the disease.
2. I will get a lot of aggressive chemo.
3. My doc will retest the BRAC gene to make sure it wasn't a false negative since that would impact my treatment.
4. I get to go back to have a port catheter installed before I can receive my chemo since the drugs are so toxic they will burn through the puny veins on the arms and must go straight into the heart. (I'm glad I didn't hear that part.)
5. I need to have a heart echocardiogram since the chemo drugs can damage the heart, so we need to check that mine is strong enough for the drugs.
6. I need to attend "chemo class" at the cancer center to find out the joys ahead of me.

7. I need to take some more Percoset or Xanax or both because I wasn't feeling too good. (The doctor didn't actually say that part. I added it.)

8. And someone needed to give my mom some drugs too since she looked like she was about to cry. (I added that part too.)

A good friend of mine I had known since junior high school called me a few weeks after my initial diagnosis. We cried together on the phone and I told him I was scared.

"But, I'm so glad it's me and not the kids," I managed to get out between sobs. "That makes it more bearable."

"You know that's why it's so hard on your folks. They wish it were them instead of you," he said quietly. We both cried harder.

A good friend later helped me see the reality that I don't have 365 bad days ahead of me. Instead, I have 4 bad days, followed by 10 good days, then 4 more bad days, then more good days, then 3 bad days followed by 4 good days and on and on.

I pushed for the double mastectomy and wanted chemo on the first visit to the oncologist, so I was prepared for a long and hard path. Why get too upset when the doc told me it would be long and hard? 15 months of chemo, possible radiation and lots of surgery.

Day 32

"Valentine, party of six," a friend announced to the receptionist when my posse showed up for Chemo Class.

I was completely shocked at the number of people attending with me. I didn't want to go myself, let alone go to someone else's Chemo Class.

It reminded me of my mother-in-law, who showed up with Greg's father at the hospital when I was in labor with our first child.

My mother was in the room with me and motioned for my mother-in-law to join us when they knocked on the door to see how far along I was.

My mother-in-law replied, "oh heavens no, I'll wait out here. I didn't want to be in the room when I gave birth myself, let alone be in the room for someone else's."

I didn't want to be in Chemo Class; I can't imagine anyone else wanting to be there either.

"Can I just get the Cliff's Notes?" I joked to my husband. He just looked at me.

I think my ostrich version of not knowing too much too soon was working for me. What if I learned something in Chemo Class about some possible side effect that I didn't even know was possible? Would I psychosomatically develop that nasty side effect once I learned about it? Nausea and fatigue are bad enough, and I was pretty content to expect those side effects.

I told my husband before Chemo Class, "You know, I was always a good and competitive student, so I expect I will want to excel at Chemo Class and get an A."

His reply: "I think in the cancer world, an 'A' is just showing up."

On the whole, the class depressed me, but seemed informative and helpful for my friends and family. My initial round of four treatments over three months would be about four hours in the "chair" hooked up to the IV drip of medicine each time. Greg pointed out that there would be warmed blankets (my favorite) and a crushed ice machine in the chemo room, so those would be my highlights of the experience.

The main lesson I took away from Chemo Class was the importance of staying hydrated. Food wasn't really as important as liquids. There would be tons of good nausea medicines, so I didn't think that will be much of a concern. Fatigue would be a big problem, but I'd been expecting that.

"There are some additional potential side effects of the typical breast cancer chemo drugs," said the oncology nurse leading the class. "Some women's fingernails turn black and even fall off."

Did I really need to hear that? Was that really helpful?

"Also, our breast cancer patients will lose their hair, eyebrows and eyelashes, but they will still need to shave their legs," the nurse added. She then commented, "this seems most unfair to me." The injustice of it all!

The reality would be actually much different. Not only did the hair on my head and face fall out, but all the hair on my body did as well. I got a full Brazilian without the pain of waxing or laser hair removal. But, the cost was high.

The chemo class continued with helpful and interesting information.

"For five days after each chemotherapy treatment, all bodily fluids would be considered hazardous waste, so everyone would have to flush the toilet twice and wear rubber gloves for any clothes that are contaminated by vomit for example," the nurse said.

Blah, blah, blah.

Somewhere along the line I stopped hearing words again so it was good that I brought a posse who hopefully were a bit less freaked out than me and were actually listening.

I returned home to find that my deacon from church had dropped off a musical singing card that congratulated me for graduating from Chemo Class! That was a lighthearted break from the awful world of fingernails falling off and hazardous waste pee.

Day 33

"You're not supposed to have an IV in the arm because you've had lymph nodes removed on both sides," the pre-op nurse informed me on the morning of my port catheter installation.

"We're going to try putting in your foot instead."

What? What new hell was this?

She called in the nurse anesthetist who attempted and failed. The anesthesiologist came in and made yet another attempt, failing also.

"Perhaps we could try a neck IV instead?" the nurse anesthetist asked the physician.

"No, no, let's keep trying the feet," I said, choosing my poison.

Finally, the doctor made the decision that an IV in the hand wouldn't be that bad and they were able to get an IV in my hand on the first try. Whew!

On a physical note, I'd felt since my initial mastectomy that I had a tight underwire bra on and couldn't wait to get it off. Of course, I couldn't. Sometimes that discomfort moved into pain but with the pain meds, usually it was just different levels of discomfort.

With the surgical port procedure, I initially felt like I had worked out my pectoral muscles and the left side was strained or unusually tired. I fell asleep at home in the afternoon and woke feeling like I was unable to even move my left upper body. I had to walk around the house holding my left arm with my right arm because I couldn't even support that arm where the port had been installed in the chest. I was hoping a good night's sleep and a bundle of medication would help the next day be better.

True to most difficult things in life, the next day was better.

I don't like the thought that there might be microscopic cancer seeds floating around in my body looking for a home, so I'm spending time telling them to leave.

Day 37

"I've seen about 50 cancer patients who were on the same chemo drugs you'll be taking," says the radiology tech as he prepared me for my baseline echocardiogram. "None of them had heart damage even though it's a possibility with that harsh drug."

I guess that was encouraging news?

My oncologist had said that there was a one percent chance of cardiac problems with the andromyacin, also known as the "red devil." Great. It wouldn't be the cancer that would get me, it would be cardiac arrest or swine flu!

Later that summer, the main side effect of one of my chemo drugs would be flu-like symptoms — fever, body aches and chills. I would wonder if I was Typhoid Mary with the actual Swine Flu or just having chemo side effects.

"If I actually get Swine Flu and die, you are not allowed to say I died of Swine Flu," I instructed my husband. "Complications due to breast cancer or something along those lines. I would die of embarrassment if my obituary says I died of Swine Flu. Of course, I'll already be dead, but you know what I mean!"

Greg and I also met yesterday with the oncologist for a final chat before the chemo began that Thursday.

"You have a "good" kind of breast cancer that's triple positive for the hormone receptors, (estrogen, progesterone and something called Her2Neu) which means there are more drugs and treatments available."

My oncologist gave me a 90 percent chance of being around in 10 years.

Not the odds I'd prefer since I intend to be here 40 more years, but 10 would be a good start. Of course, Dr. K said that he has no way of knowing if I'm the 90 or 10 percent category of the odds he quoted.

"So, there's a 10 percent chance of me dying before then?" I asked.

"Well, not really," my doctor explained. "Your odds are really 100 percent or 0 percent. We just don't know which patients are the 100 percent and which ones are the 0 percent."

"Yes, well the 10 percent chance of dying is really because of my increased risk of a traffic fatality since being diagnosed with cancer means I'll be on the road twice a week traveling to and from the oncology office," I said.

Being diagnosed with cancer is not only scary, but it's inconvenient. Patients spend more time in the oncologist's office, getting lab work and chemo and exams and scans...it really interferes with "real" life.

Dr. K also said he discussed my case with some MD Anderson trained colleagues who had differing opinions on the treatment. Basically, there are the ACT and TAC camps of treatment. It's the order the chemo drugs are given and the drugs themselves. Some docs prefer to leave out the regimen I'm about to do because of that one percent chance of heart problems.

Dr. K and one MD Anderson friend prefer to include that drug because of a risk of recurrence. Since I'm young, with no heart problems, Dr. K thinks it would be worth taking the heart risk.

Day 42

"I know how cancer is going to kill me," I commented to a friend after my first chemotherapy. "It's going to bore me to death."

"Seriously, Amy..." Julie replies, laughing at my description of the rather boring eight-hour ordeal.

"The most uncomfortable part of the experience was knowing that there was poison seeping into my body through the infusion tubes."

"Yes, but aren't antibiotics a form of poison? Alcohol too?" she replies. "You don't seem too upset when you had to take drugs for strep throat or had a second beer at my house."

"Okay, but still!

The day after my first chemo treatment I spent the whole day mostly horizontal, trying to ward off any potential nausea... Late in the afternoon, I got up and was a bit more of my usual self. I realized that a month of infirmity is about my limit. I wanted to do things and be with people and get on with it.

But my body might not cooperate.

"I'm frustrated!" I complained to my husband. "The novelty of having cancer has worn off."

Amy K. brought me some medicine and stayed for dinner, and then Paul and Dino showed up to help me get the kids bathed and to bed since Greg had a one day trip to Amarillo. The kids were delighted to find out he had to take 4 airplanes in one day. It was lovely having company over and they were a great help with the ordinary tasks of dinner and bedtime.

My nausea had been under control until about 1 a.m., when my usual chest pain started. Since my stomach seemed a bit queasy, I was reluctant to take my pain meds and muscle relaxers. After one Saltine (my morning sickness savior), I decided to risk the drugs and am happy I did, because the nausea seemed to have subsided as my chest pain decreased.

"It's the reconstruction expanders under my pec muscles that are causing me the continual pain," I told my friend Di later that week. "If I had I elected not to do the reconstruction, I would be over the worst of the surgery."

However, I never thought twice about the reconstruction because in my mind, I was going to live another 40 years and having breasts seemed a natural part of that lifespan.

"Did you ever think of not doing the reconstruction?" she asked.

"No. Being a small-breasted woman to begin with, I've padded enough bras as a teen. I didn't want to wear special padded bras for 40 years."

And just think how good I was going to look in a bathing suit in a year. Or two.

Day 44

"Do you know if you will die before me?" my four-year old Daniel asked.

"No," I had to answer. "I don't know that, but I have a pretty good idea since most parents die before their children."

I know we'd had these conversations before my illness, so there was nothing unusual about it. The timeframe is always interesting because to four-year-old Daniel, one year or five years or forty years seem the same. He is still trying to understand the relationship between yesterday, today and tomorrow, so anything beyond that seems like eons. And Sara is very goth and dramatic in her outlook, and proclaims that we're all going to die in one second or one minute, and counts down the time. However, the conversation was especially poignant to me in light of the unwelcome bodily guests supposedly floating through my lymphatic system.

Day 46

Women out there will appreciate the irony of this post; the men may prefer to ignore it. One of the joys of chemotherapy is that the drugs will throw my body into menopause 10 years earlier than expected. My body is obviously confused and the universe is unusually cruel: this morning at Sara's elementary school, I took off my floppy hat to fan myself and realized I was having my period and a hot flash at the same time. Seriously, how can I not laugh about this?

Day 48

As my emotions are heightened with my drug-induced mania and my constant thoughts of cancer taking me away from my husband and children, I renew friendships through Facebook and email, discovering that people feel the need to express their heartfelt emotions to me in case I die. Later, I realized that I hadn't spoken or seen many of these friends for years, and might not have had any contact with them again in my life if it hadn't been for the cancer.

I stayed up late at night reminiscing with old friends, until my husband rolled his eyes and told me to leave these poor folks alone. I think he thought I was stalking ex-boyfriends and long-lost friends. Perhaps I was. This behavior was unlike the straight-laced Amy I had been. I had always followed the rules and walked a narrow path. I never stayed out past curfew, never cheated on a boyfriend, never shoplifted lipstick from a drugstore. I began email conversations with ex boyfriends and even ran a stop sign in the middle of the night when no one was around. The Amy I had been who always followed the rules had gotten cancer. Maybe this new rebellious Amy wouldn't.

My oncologist said, "Most people would be under the table at this point."

I gave him a weak smile. "Is that really an option?"

Where's the table? I wanted under it.

I think I'm just too practical to do much besides put one foot in front of the other. A friend told me that in some situations in life, you can sidestep around things. Other times, you must go straight through. I think she was right about this one. This is one of those times when you have to move straight through. One step at a time.

Day 51

"Really? No, *really?*" I asked Doctor H. (my plastic surgeon). He filled a syringe with what looked like a lot of saline and started towards my naked torso.

"Don't I get novocaine or something?" I asked in a slightly panicky voice, as he proceeded to feel my chest and the top of my expanders, looking for the opening in the plastic bag expander under the skin to inject the saline.

"No, your chest is still numb from the surgery," he said, as he inserted the needle into my upper breast. "You won't feel anything."

And he was right.

My breast slowly inflated as he injected the saline. I looked like that doll in the Barbie family I had in the 70s. I think her name was "Grow Up Jody" or something. You turned the doll's arm and her chest would expand as if she were developing breasts as a teen.

Dr. H explained, "I was able to put some saline into the expanders when I first put them in your body during the mastectomy so we will inject the saline every three weeks two or three more times until we're the size we want."

"Please, no stripper boobs," I begged my plastic surgeon.

Dr. H said, "No stripper boobs. Trust me. I've done this before and will get you to a size that will look natural with the rest of your body."

"Can I amend my previous statement?" I asked, after thinking a bit longer. "Maybe a little bigger than I was – very small stripper boobs."

Apparently, I can't really be as small as I had started since the implants don't come in an A cup size. My eventual final size will also be determined by how much the pec muscles and skin will stretch during the expander process. It's not as easy as a woman getting a "boob job" to increase her breast size.

Day 53

I'm learning so much about my cancer and chemo treatments! After my lab work, I chatted with the nurse practitioner and she brought in Dr. K to discuss my genetic tests. The doctors are all so happy that my first treatment went well, with relatively few side effects (according to them), and my blood work still looks good.

There was one bad night/morning and then a few bad half days. The oncologists adjusted my chemo treatment and anti-nausea meds to make the next round a bit better.

The two drug cocktail I take now hit the invisible and supposed cancer cells at different times in their growth cycle. Researchers have figured out the exact timeframe and amount of the drugs in my mix to kill any remaining cancer in my body. I never realized that my white and red blood cells don't need to drop in order for the chemo to work. That's just an unfortunate byproduct of the chemo, and the docs can manipulate my meds to increase my cell counts if I need it. That's why the weekly lab work is so important. And the chemo doesn't stay in my body for three weeks fighting the cancer. It kills what it needs to kill during the first few hours, and then the docs want you to flush the chemicals from your body with lots of liquids to keep the drugs from hurting the good cells. It usually takes a few days to get the drugs out of your body, so by now, I'm probably chemical-free, which is a good feeling.

So, I can look at these first four treatments as one potential bad day after each treatment, and a few more sick half days along the way, then a week or two of good days until the next treatment. Since I'm through one treatment, that's only three more bad days and maybe nine bad half days ahead of me. I just might be able to do that! There is a cumulative effect of the treatments, so the last one is worse than the first one, simply because your body is more tired from being bombarded with nasty chemicals. But, I think I can make it if there are only three more bad treatments. After the Adromyacin, the next round of Taxol chemo doesn't include nausea as a side effect, so most people prefer it to this round.

Since my usually good insurance company won't pay for a second round of genetic testing, the nurse practitioner asked Dr. K to discuss the importance of having this test done. They all agreed we can wait a while to make that decision. I wanted to make sure I wasn't going to contract ovarian cancer in the next year while we're waiting to do that genetic test.

They all laughed and assured me I wasn't getting cancer in the next few years with all the drugs in my body.

I have three months of this first round of drugs, three months of a second round, then we move to six months of "targeted" drug therapy since I'm lucky enough to have triple positive hormone receptor tumors. Then, we have five years of hormone treatment with Tamoxifen, which isn't even an infusion just a daily pill. After that, we have five years of additional hormone treatment to keep my estrogen levels low.

Of course, some bodies and some cancers don't respond well to the drugs, and the chemicals themselves have nasty side effects. All of that can lead to an early demise, but as the nurse practitioner said, "the world of breast cancer research is changing so rapidly that who knows what remarkable drugs and treatments we will have in five or ten years?"

Day 60

Most people walk around with white blood cell counts between 4,500 and 10,000. Mine are now 700. Wow. I'm a bit depressed because this was my first chemotherapy treatment, and I was supposedly the strongest I was going to be going into this whole kit and kaboodle. I'm tired and not feeling great, but I assumed since I had surgery 6 weeks ago and chemo 2 weeks ago, that feeling poorly was just part of the deal. So, I just have to wait until my white blood cells are reborn, then they get hit again by the next chemo. Don't cough around me, please.

Day 62

Today I saw an energy healer and an acupuncturist to keep me emotionally and physically strong while undergoing chemo. Let's see, next week I have a plastic surgeon appointment on Monday, a *Wonders and Worries* appointment on Tuesday to discuss psychological support for our kids while Mommy gets well, and another acupuncturist appointment on Wednesday in time to strengthen my immune system for the Thursday chemo onslaught. This getting well is getting exhausting!

Day 64

Cancer is unruly and misbehaved and messes with my family, which angers me. Of course, some of that is Greg and my decision not to hide my medical condition from the children, so they hear about the cancer and treatments. We try to hide the stress and fear, but the reality is that stress comes out whether or not a family chooses to maintain open communication about the disease.

One evening we were all playing UNO Attack, card game where an electronic dealing machine randomly spits out cards to the players, giving them a random disadvantage in the game.

After I had not received any cards for a few turns, Sara commented, "Maybe the machine knows that Mommy has breast cancer."

Sara came home from school last week saying she and a gaggle of girls in first grade were planning on creating a Rock Band. She wanted the musicians to wear an assortment of my wigs for their concerts. I'm sure the other girls were wondering why Sara's mom has an assortment of wigs.

The most dramatic moment was earlier this week when I was taking Daniel to a play date so I could go to a lab appointment. While driving there, I asked him, "do you think Mommy would rather go to the doctor or to your play date with you?"

Daniel immediately said, "The doctor's!" Since everything Daniel says has an exclamation point at the end, it sounded like I was particularly enthusiastic about my doctor's visit.

I said, "no, I'd rather go to play," because I fear the kids think I prefer all these doctor's visits to spending time with them.

Daniel replied, "No, you want to go to the doctor's because he's making you well!" Again, with the enthusiastic exclamation point.

Sara, who does not always forge an easy path for herself without cancer in her life, has so much anger and grumpiness these days. Daniel has thrown two major temper tantrums with literal red-faced screaming and wild thrashing and kicking in the past week. Not that Sara wouldn't be angry or grumpy on her own, or Daniel wouldn't throw a temper tantrum since he is four, but I know my children's normal behavior patterns and personalities. Both of them are showing the stress of this situation and all I feel is anger that the damned cancer is hurting my children.

Do what you want to me, but leave my children alone!

Day 65

I run my fingers through my short hair and get handfuls of loose strands. My hair is thick enough that it's not noticeably showing, but I know this is the beginning. It's irritating because I feel like I'm cat shedding, leaving blond strands on the pillow, in the shower, on my clothes. At least it's starting to happen. Maybe Greg will clip me into a crew cut this weekend. A fellow cancer patient told me she clipped her hair into a buzz cut, then ran a sticky lint roller over her head each day. More and more hair came off until she was bald. That sounds like the way to go.

I was starting to think if my hair didn't start falling out soon, I'd need another haircut. That seemed a bit ridiculous, considering…

Day 66

Strange what dates we commemorate while others, equally important, pass by invisible and unnoticed. The dates that stand out in my life always seemed to be happy before March 2009 — birthdays, anniversaries, holidays. But after March 27th, the remarkable dates all have a somber note.

In my happier past, I could tell you the day I married Greg, but not the date I fell in love with him. I could tell you the birthdays of both our children, but not the dates they were conceived. More recently, I could tell you the date a doctor told me I had cancer, but not the date the first cell forgot to die. I can list the dates of my biopsy, my surgery, my first chemo treatment, but will never be able to celebrate the exact day that the last cancer cell in my body died. Eventually, I will be able to commemorate my last A/C infusion, my last Taxol infusion, my last Herceptin infusion, my last Tamoxifen pill, but will never know the date at which I became "cancer-free." I choose to assume I am already liberated from my misbehaving ductal cells but who really knows?

So, one more date to add to my growing list of cancer-related days to remember: May 31st, the day I shaved my head as the hair began to fall out. This one isn't so bad — I only cried a little when the hairstylist gifted the buzz cut to me instead of accepting payment. And I won't count the tears that fell due to someone's kindness, because those are much better than the days I cry due to my own self-pity or discomfort or fear of the unknown. With my penchant for looking at the past with rose-hued glasses, I suspect I will forget the actual dates of my cancer diagnosis, my double mastectomy, my chemotherapy. These will all be lumped into that rough patch way back in 2009-2010.

While I may forget the actual date, I probably will remember my husband trying to pay my hairstylist Vanessa at funky Bird's Barbershop and hearing her yell back, "No, no, no, this one is no charge. This is my gift."

Day 70

Finished the second of many chemo treatments.

I didn't want to go there, be there, or even think about it. It's really not bad because I have the chest port, so don't even feel a stick so I can't complain about the pain. It's knowing that I'm pouring toxic chemicals into my body, albeit for a good cause. And the dread of what side effects may follow. The drugs themselves gave me a sinus headache during infusion, so the nurses slowed down my drip. We had a bit of delay because the CBC (complete blood count) machine was broken so my pre-infusion blood test had to be driven down to the south location of Texas Oncology. Every time I am scheduled for infusion, my blood has to be tested because if my cell counts are too low, making me too weak for the strong medicine, the chemo will be rescheduled. That's why I don't have any definite chemo dates on my calendar in the future. For those of you counting, my white blood cell had dropped to 700 but was 3,500 on infusion day. That's still low, and I'll probably never reach my pre-chemo treatment high of 4,500, but it was high enough for the infusion to happen. So now I wait, take my anti-nausea meds which make me sleepy, and my steroid, which hypes me up. With my competing internal pharmacy, I'm not sure if I'm tired or wired.

My folks are here and are a huge help, entertaining the kids and helping with meal prep. I have to thank all my friends for their support in bringing me meals, commenting on my blogs (receiving that feedback means so much), taking the kids for play dates, or just keeping me and my family in their prayers. And Greg doesn't get much credit, but he is my rock in all of this. A few folks have asked about him, knowing how hard the role of caregiver is. Before my infusion, I apologized to my nurse that I was in such a bitchy mood. She said I seemed perky, happy, and fine. I turned to Greg and he diplomatically said, "no comment," because he had to put up with my pre-infusion anxiety, calming my fears with his quiet presence.

Day 71

Two days after my second chemo infusion, a mosquito landed on my arm. I watched it, about to slap it away, when it decided my blood smelled strange and flew away on its own accord. My blood is no longer sweet to the mosquitoes. I guess I'll take my blessings where I find them these strange days.

Day 72

This round of chemo's side effects haven't been that bad. I'm very grateful and appreciative, although I don't feel great. I feel like I'm on the verge of getting sick, having a bad headache or stomachache, but nothing ever materializes. The oncologist gave me steroid pills along with the two crazy-strong anti-nausea drugs. I'm part wired and part tired. Now that I'm off the steroid, I'm starting to crash.

Day 75

Still doing okay after my second chemo ... but if this is what good feels like, I'm grateful I've avoided bad. I'm a wimp when it comes to illnesses because I've never had a sickness that made me feel bad for more than a week. I think I can remember having bronchitis my freshman year of college and a high-fever flu when I first moved to Austin. Other than that, all my illnesses have been the garden-variety colds, sore throats, or stomach aches that came and went without much notice. So, to not feel well, but not exactly be sick, is tiring and frustrating and annoying, because I know the nasty effects the systemic chemo is having on my whole body. I have the start of a headache, the start of nausea, intestinal discomfort, chills and fatigue, but none of it moves past the annoying stage to the really sick stage. I think once I begin the targeted Herceptin, which attacks the cancer cells themselves, I'll mentally feel better. I have never liked taking medicine for no reason; killing off all fast-growing cells in my body seems like placing some unnecessary sacrifices upon my poor body in this war against cancer. And for probably the first time in my life, I have an actual good reason to say that I'm officially depressed. The irony is, that new studies show that common anti-depressants like Zoloft and Prozac have been shown to reduce the effectiveness of breast cancer chemotherapy regimens. At least that conundrum amuses me and reminds me of God's funny sense of humor.

Day 77

Today, I took Sara to the eye doctor for her annual exam. She chose darling hot pink glasses and is quite thrilled with them. I was going to wear a wig, but the kids wanted me just to wear a hat, so I chose to accessorize with my jaunty brown newsboy cap, which keeps my head warm but doesn't really disguise the fact that I have lost my hair.

The doctor was very interested in my cancer, so we discussed it at some length.

At the end of the visit, the doctor asked, "How long has it been since your last eye exam?"

I explained, "I'm overdue for one, but an eye exam is low on my medical to-do list these days."

"I recommend you get one soon because breast cancer likes to metastasize to the back of the eye. I've actually seen a patient with that."

What???? Breast cancer of the eyeball? I know I might not be taking this very seriously, but if I really got breast cancer of the eyeball, I think I would burst out laughing. It just sounds like a bad B-movie at this point! I'll chat with my oncologist tomorrow and keep everyone up to date on the health and wellbeing of my eyeballs.

Day 78

I know my friends and relatives are on pins and needles waiting to see what my oncologist thinks about my potential for breast cancer of the eyeball. He very quickly determined that breast cancer of the eyeball is among the least of my worries.

"Are you having any vision problems?" my doctor asked.

"No, but does breast cancer like to metastasize to the back of the eyeball?"

"Cancer can spread to anywhere in the body," he answered, "but I don't usually order eye exams for my breast cancer patients unless they are having vision problems because it's not a usual place that the cancer will spread first."

"I think it's unlikely you have eyeball cancer," he finished.

My friend Amy K. came with me and had some hilarious comments about optometrists.

"I think optometrists might be at the bottom of the medical doctor totem pole and they are dying to prove themselves by diagnosing strange and rare diseases," she said. "I once saw an optometrist who scared me into thinking I had diabetes from something she saw in my eye exam."

Whew, my eyeballs seem safe for now. But...there is always more fun in my cancer world. Since I had a migraine type headache after both A/C chemo treatments, my oncologist wants me to have an MRI brain scan to make sure the headaches are simply drug-related, and not a sign of something worse. Please someone, make the fun stop...

It's good to have friends.

Day 79

My friend Bryce relieved my troubled mind about the brain MRI. He sent me an email stating that the doctors weren't looking for brain metastasis with the MRI, rather they're looking for chemo-induced encephalitis, which is easily treatable. Bryce is a lawyer and not a doctor, yet it sounded like a plausible technical answer, so I queried him further.

"A doctor friend gave me that information," he said.

I thanked them both, then thought I'd check the doctor's credentials, given the latest "breast cancer of the eyeball" scare.

"So, what kind of doctor is this friend of yours? An optometrist by chance?"

Bryce sent a one-word email, which completely banished all doubt as to the credibility of the medical information.

"Neurosurgeon."

Day 82

Neutropenic again. This time my white blood cell count is 300. Just as a reminder: normal range is 4,500 to 10,000. I feel fine considering I'm on the verge of getting sick just from walking into the grocery store or breathing the air at the kids' Vacation Bible School. Keep your germs to yourself for a few days, please, while my blood cells recover and I take my prophylactic antibiotics.

Day 83

The brain MRI didn't happen this morning because my expanders have a form of metal in them. So, after a few phone calls, the MRI was rescheduled in favor of a brain CT. Since I was scheduled for chest and abdomen CTs tomorrow, I asked if we could just combine all three scans into one procedure. Yay — one port IV, two cups of berry-flavored barium drink, three tablespoons of flan-like paste washed down with a cup of banana flavored barium. All on an empty stomach that's already slightly queasy from last week's chemo. This time around, the contrast dye was uncomfortable instead of tickly. Sigh, I guess everything's becoming less fun. I feel like I could sleep forever.

Day 84

All scans clean! Do I need to say any more? Now I just have to deal with my regular breast cancer, instead of breast cancer of the liver, lungs or brain.

Day 85

After receiving good news on my CT scans, today seems like such a happy day. The sun is shining, people

are nice, birds are sweetly singing at the bird feeders outside our living room. It's so funny how relative happiness
is — I still have Stage III breast cancer with a long dark
road of chemotherapy ahead of me, but somehow it
doesn't seem as bad as it could be.

Day 88

Happy Birthday to Me! Happy Birthday to Me!

I'm delighted to have turned 43 today. It feels somehow more acceptable to have cancer at 43 than at 42. I've
survived another year, yay, even though it's only been
three months since my cancer diagnosis. It only seems
like a full year.

My plastic surgeon Dr. H. gave me more inflatable
boobage for my birthday.

"I like the blonde curls," he said, noticing my long
curly wig that made me look like a rock star out of the
1980s. "You seem to be doing really well during your
chemo."

"As long as I don't die, it's manageable," I said.

"That about sums it up for all of us, doesn't it." By now
Doctor H. had gotten used to my irreverent cancer attitude.

Thinking about what I just said, I amended my statement to, "Well, even if I die, I guess I'll manage that too."

But, I'm not planning on going anywhere since birthdays are so much fun. Let's all plan for 40 more!

Day 89

Sara and Daniel have learned that certain words are "bad words" in our house — "stupid" being the main one. Yesterday, Sara wanted my attention to show me a play she and her best friend had put together. I was finishing my birthday blog entry so put off Sara until I could complete my computer work.

Sara got frustrated and said, "is this what happens when you get stupid cancer? You have to type on the computer and can't come see our play right away?"

I automatically replied, "Sara, don't use the word stupid."

Sara looked at me, and I swear I saw an old, wise woman staring at me out of her eyes as she said, "But cancer *is* stupid Mommy. I think that's a good use of the word."

Yes, Sara, you can use "stupid" when you're talking about cancer because it is very, very stupid.

Day 90

Today at *Wonders and Worries*, a counseling service for children whose parents have a life-threatening disease, the children made Feelings Gardens. Sara came out of her play therapy session with a flower pot she decorated that had paper flowers sticking out of it, each one representing a different emotion. These were feelings Sara has had since finding out that her Mommy has cancer. They included some obvious, and some surprising flowers: sad, angry, frustrated, exhausted, jealous, bored, confident, smug, and the biggest flower of all was hopeful. Sara and I chatted about why she felt each emotion while Daniel had his turn to create a feelings garden. When he came out of the playroom, his flowerpot had only one large flower: sad.

Day 91

Despite my strong desire to avoid today's chemo and just keep driving south on I-35, all the way to Mexico City or Panama or wherever I-35 would take me, I made it to my oncologist office this morning. That might be due to the fact that Greg was driving and made sure I made it to the church on time, or the fact that I took a Xanax earlier that morning and wasn't quite so intent on not doing another treatment. After drawing my blood for the requisite lab work, Dr. K told me my white blood cell counts have recovered from their low of 300 last week. I'm at 6000! Unbelievable! The nurses had told me I probably wouldn't reach my pre-chemo high of 4,500 because of the treatment. Dr. K said it's because of my "clean living" and the fact that I'm young, strong and healthy. The chemo is still working at killing any stray cancer cells, despite the fact that I still have blonde peach fuzz on my head, eyebrows and a high white blood cell count. I'm not feeling great physically, but mentally I'm in the game to win it. It's nice when your healthy condition makes your usually dour oncologist smile.

Day 92

Could the third chemo be easier than the first two? So far, so good.

On an everyday basis, I need to watch my words because the day before chemo, I ran into a friend I haven't seen for a while. She'd been keeping up with my blog and was understandably concerned about my day-to-day health. That was one of the afternoons when the heat reached 103 degrees and I had been running errands with the kids, so was feeling extremely hot. My friend said something about the weather being so hot and I replied, "I know, I'm dying!" She took it in a health-related way instead of a heat-related way, and told another friend how worried she was about me. When the miscommunication was cleared up, we all laughed about it, but I need to watch my language from now on. So, if the grapevine has reached you that I'm dying, you can rest easy.

Day 103

The fifth day after chemo has been one of my hardest for the past two treatments, so I was grateful that today had been easier. I felt like I had a cold or sinus infection, but didn't have the nasty headache that prompted my oncologist to order the scary round of brain scans. Knowing my doctor's penchant for checking everything out with a thorough scan, I was a bit concerned about mentioning every little symptom to him, although he did scoff a bit at the "breast cancer of the eyeball" scare, so perhaps I can mention my cold symptoms to him without fear. Is it just my cancer diagnosis or does everyone have a sneaking suspicion that the things one mocks will come back and bite them? Whenever I laugh about eyeball cancer, I think that I'm bound to get eyeball cancer just because I'm laughing at the absurdity of it. Really, is any cancer not absurd?

Sara told her first grade teacher that "Mommy has too much breasts," when I was first diagnosed. I think Mrs. H looked at my slender figure and tried to look serious while wanting to smile at the puzzling image of me having "too many breasts."

Sara was technically correct in that many cells in my breasts had forgotten to die and were crowding together where they no longer needed to be. I prefer to think of the cancer cells as misguided and confused, rather than aggressive and invasive, which are the adjectives doctors use to describe my illness.

So, in the quest to use the proper language to describe my condition, I prefer to say "I had breast cancer," instead of "have" breast cancer. It may be a small point, but since the experts can't tell me whether or not I still have cancer in my body, I prefer the past tense. And if there are any misguided cells still in my body, I prefer to think that my strong and healthy immune system, along with the onslaught of perfectly timed nasty chemo drugs, will convince those confused cells of their mortality and sweep them from my body.

Day 105

Happy 49th Anniversary Mom and Dad! Greg and I will celebrate our 9th wedding anniversary this fall. Funny how all those milestones seem to mean more these days.

I've been delighted that this round of chemo hasn't been as bad as the first two.

Day 112

To keep everyone up to date on the joys of my immune system being torn down from the chemo, I have a summer cold, messed up sinuses and tiny red sores on the inside of my mouth. My throat started to hurt the day before, and it felt like the sores were in the back of my throat. Does that mean they now line my intestinal tract too? Yuck. A little salt water/baking soda gargle made everything more comfortable and a good night's sleep helped too. Today, I've slowly felt better as the day progressed. Probably more white blood cells are flooding my system, helping to normalize my entire intestinal tract and mucus membranes, since those are the areas my chemo affects the most. I'm not running a fever, so as long as I avoid the swine flu while my system is shot, I'll make it. It's uncomfortable and irritating and frustrating, but if the chemo is killing any remaining cancer, I'll manage. I don't want to write, I can't think of anything funny, it all seems hard, so I just put one foot in front of the other. I'm sure tomorrow will be a better day since today was so much better than yesterday.

Day 115 to 153

Day 115

Tomorrow is another trip to the hellish land of chemo. All in all, I know the chemo is not that bad, despite my complete and total dislike of my port being drawn for the lab and drugs. When the nurses put the needle into the chest port, the patient gets a "skunk smell" in their skull that permeates the nose and mouth.

I know my side effects are controlled by strong and serious pharmaceuticals. (Wired and tired at the same time due to conflicting anti-nausea and steroid drugs...)

I know the drugs are poisoning any remaining cancer. (If there is even any cancer left in my body...) I know the nausea, fatigue, sinus problems, intestinal discomfort, mouth sores, and low white blood counts are temporary. (Please God, make them temporary...)

I know I'm less of a wuss about medical stuff than folks I hear of who can't stand the sight of blood, or faint when they see needles or have a low threshold for pain. (May no one with a weak stomach ever get cancer...)

I know all of this, but I'm still a mess dreading my chemo day. Greg reminded me that "everyone says tomorrow is the last of the hard ones." I started crying and said, "easy for everyone else to say – they don't have to do the chemo."

Day 116

The last of the "hard" chemos is behind me. This time, I began to feel bad during the drip, so wonderful Nurse Rachel popped some Atavan in the medicine. It took away some of the nausea and left me with a Valium calming buzz. I'm still peeing red, which means the ultra nasty Andromiacin is still in my system. My instructions are to flush the toilet twice after peeing, although Dr. K laughed a bit and said that's more to protect the dog who might be drinking from the toilet than the rest of the household family members.

I get another echo in two weeks to double check my heart's health. Then, while I'm on the Herceptin, I'll receive regular echoes every three months, since that drug is also hard on the heart. My next round of drugs is a weekly Taxol/Herceptin combination for 12 weeks, and then I move into my pure Herceptin round for 51 weeks. I'm not feeling great, and will probably spend most of the weekend in bed or lazing around the house.

Thank God for wonderful caregivers like my mother-in-law Carol who is here to help, and my friends who sweetly and routinely drop off food at the house. My folks have been here for surgeries and other chemo treatments, and volunteered to take care of kids at a moment's notice, especially last week when I wasn't feeling well. Greg's been putting the kids to bed and getting them food when I'm exhausted at the end of the day.

So far, so good. I'm feeling fine, and halved my steroid pill so haven't been as wired as last time. With the last chemo, my alternate side effects hit me a week to 10 days later when the dry sinuses, mouth sores and fatigue hit, so I guess I'll wait and see. I'm going to sleep soon with maybe a Phernegan pill to knock me out and give me a good night's rest.

On a funnier note, Daniel told me he thinks I'll live to be 108. I told him that would be great and he'd be 70 when I'm 108, which gave him belly laughs because that was so funny. I'm sure he never thought about being as old as his grandparents. Ever!

Day 119

It's a world of ups and downs. I started out feeling fine, but wore down slowly as the day continued. It's hard to say exactly what's wrong — I just don't feel right, and some of that is due to the fact that there are conflicting pharmaceuticals in my system. My intestinal tract isn't fine, and I'm not nauseated and still eating, but the thought of food turns me off. I'm tired and wired and not sure if my body wants to sleep or stay up. I'm in turns happy and weepy and down. I want to feel better and spend time with the kids because I'm scared I have a limited amount of time. Even if it's reduced from 40 years to 30 years, I feel the need to maximize every moment. Yet, I'm tired and depressed and just want to escape this strange world for a drugged sleep. My bladder is a bit irritated by the chemo, so I'm chugging cranberry juice and my skin is dry so I'm slathering on the lotion. Now I'm just rambling again – due to the steroids I'm sure – but this blog is probably describing the conflicting internal emotions and physical feelings accurately, even if it is hard to understand.

Day 121

"Why don't you believe that you are one of the many breast cancer patients who doesn't even need the chemo because of the nature of your tumors," suggested my acupuncturist.

"The regimen is good and outcomes are in your favor," he continued.

If we believe the clinical data, up to 50 percent of all breast cancer patients, even Stage IIIA, don't need chemo to live a long and healthy life cancer-free. But everyone gets hit by the poison, because medical science hasn't figured out who is which half of the 50 percent. While that sounds positive and encouraging, the how of it still mystifies me.

How do I believe there is no cancer remaining in my body when I feel like my body and mind are falling apart due to the drugs? How do I remain positive and encouraged when my children are at each other's throats at the slightest hint that Mommy is not her usual strong self? How do I have the energy to continue my weekly schedule of blood withdrawals, doctor visits, echocardiograms, chemo infusions, surgeries, diagnostic scans, acupuncture appointments, and *Wonders and Worries* child therapy visits when I still have 52 weeks ahead of me?

"Okay, I will," I tell my acupuncturist. "But it's hard enough when your body is strong before the chemo hits and your mind is still unscathed by the steroids and chemo-brain…but now? It's hard to believe."

Daunting is the best word, yet I'm not even sure about my vocabulary anymore since I'm so addle-brained. Maybe the best word is "discouraging" or "difficult" or "challenging" or that particular word which escapes me right now, but is just outside my train of thought…

Day 124

The reality dance competition *So You Think You Can Dance* featured a tribute to a woman fighting breast cancer. The female dancer wore a purple head scarf and threw herself around the stage in a too-familiar barrage of roller coaster emotions while being supported by her strong male partner. It was very touching and inspirational, and prompted several phone calls and email messages from friends. I even wore my purple head scarf yesterday in tribute to the wonderful dance. Sara had heard about the dance from me, and also from various friends commenting on it throughout the day.

She saw a brief recap of the performance before bedtime last night and commented in her logical, matter-of-fact way, "I don't think a woman who really had breast cancer would be able to jump around the stage like that. She wouldn't have all that energy or feel like leaping into the air." No one's pulling any wool over this seven-year-old's eyes!

Day 127

Part of my surreal world these days is my "staged breast reconstruction." Today was my last saline fill-up in preparation for the eventual soft gel implants. I've been visiting the relaxing spa-like atmosphere of my plastic surgeon's office every two or three weeks for the last four months, so I will miss those regular appointments. Each time, the surgeon inserts a needle through my pec muscles and injects approximately 2 oz. of saline into the expanders, which fill up like water balloons under my chest. For my relatives and friends who have accompanied me to the visits, it's been a wild experience watching my chest expand. Someone asked me if it felt like having my braces tightened when I was a teen. Similar...very similar. Dr. H told Greg and me today that I have approximately 13 oz. of fluid in each side. If you imagine a Coke can containing 12 ounces, you get an idea of the volume.

Since the saline is contained in the plastic expanders under my pec muscles, the description of a Coke can is fairly accurate, both in how they feel sitting on my chest and how they feel when I touch them. In three or four months, my second surgery will take place to replace the hard plastic expanders with soft gel implants. As a funny sidebar to this whole experience, I'll be going with Greg to Washington D.C. next week on a business trip and the kids will be with my folks in Houston. I had to get a letter from my surgeon explaining about my chest expanders and portacath because both contain metal and may set off the airport metal detector.

Day 133

"I haven't been writing or calling anyone lately, because I've been crazy," I explained to a friend.

"What do you mean, "crazy?" she asked.

"Well, I've been having racing thoughts, wild emotions and I sat up for hours last night trying to figure out if thinking I was crazy really meant I was crazy – or if I wouldn't think about being crazy if I really were crazy."

"Oh, actual *crazy* crazy."

The good news was my oncology staff seemed quite comfortable with my steroid-induced mania. The nurse who accessed my chest port in preparation for my chemo noticed that I was talking very fast and in a very animated fashion.

"I'm always animated and I always talk fast," I responded, thinking she was a bit crazy herself.

"No, this is different," she said, "I think you may have a touch of steroid mania."

"I think she's right," Dr. K concurred, and suggested stepping down the steroids a bit to calm me down.

"Have you been up all night cleaning out your closets?" he asked.

"No, dammit. Why couldn't I have that kind of mania? Instead, I obsessed about finding knitting lessons for my four-year-old son when he tells me he doesn't want to return to his soccer team in the fall, and would prefer instead to do something with his hands."

This seemed very normal to me. Another mark of the crazy.

After calling a few fabric stores to inquire about children's knitting classes, a fellow mom friend says she thought Daniel was talking about a sport where you catch the ball with your hands like football or baseball. Oh, of course.

My oncologist referred me to a psychiatrist since those medical specialties help manage medication interactions that affect the brain. The medical scheduler was attempting to make an appointment, and put her hand over the mouthpiece as she was talking to the psychiatrist receptionist to ask me, "Is this for electroshock therapy?"

What!? No!

Needless to say, I decided not to see a psychiatrist and instead promised my oncologist that I'd come back if the steroid mania didn't get better in a week.

"Instead of cleaning out my closets, I spent two hours last night wondering how to spell the word "who."

"No more Dr. Seuss for you," Dr. K. said.

Day 138

Yesterday, I had my first Taxol/Herceptin drug combo. This is an infusion too, and I wound up at the oncologist's office from about 9 a.m. until 5:30, after closing. Because it was my first time to have these new drugs, the nurses drip the infusions really slowly (1 teaspoon every hour), and pump me full of allergy meds and steroids to counter any possible allergic reaction. And we're not talking rashes or hives; it's a full-blown anaphylactic shock if you're allergic to Taxol. Great fun!

My friend Amy K. was there with me and we both told Nurse Rachel how glad we were that I had a friend there in case of a reaction. Rachel said, "Oh, believe me, we all have eyes on you the whole time…" and they did. All the nurses walked by frequently, and my oncologist even stopped by to check on me. Usually he leaves me in the capable hands of the infusion nurses, and I mean capable. They recommend changing doses of medicines, adding different ones, and question the doctor on choices of pre-infusion or post-chemo meds. These are the people you want around you in a health crisis. No wilting flowers in the infusion room!

So, after my Benadryl, I start feeling sleepy. Then, I curled my legs up and started wiggling around in the chair, without really realizing I was doing it. Sure enough, Rachel comes over and says she noticed that I have "restless leg" syndrome because of the Benadryl dose. My friend Amy comments how she noticed I went from drowsy to agitated in a few moments' time. So, I get Atavan to calm me down.

Another nurse walks by and says she's glad to see my legs stretched back out. I'm impressed that the nurses are watching something so seemingly insignificant as leg position while their patients are getting the drug infusions.

My brother came to relieve Amy K. and I fell asleep. The next thing I know, Greg is waking me up and he's there with a nurse I don't know. It's past closing time and the drugs are done, so it's time to take out the needle. Future chemo infusions shouldn't be this long and involved, since I didn't have an allergic reaction.

And today, I feel pretty darn good. No nausea, just a little steroid mania, and no exceptional fatigue. Last night I had some arm/wrist tingling, which may come and go with this drug, but today my fingers are able to type, so the neuropathy hasn't set in yet. This seems like a pretty boring post to me, but these days, boring equals good.

Day 140

Damned cancer. I can feel myself getting crazier and crazier as the steroid mania starts to take over. I had four hours sleep and was up in the middle of the night with my mind racing. I stayed in bed and watched the clock change minute by minute until hours had passed. Why didn't I get up and watch *House Hunters* on HGTV or finish reading *My Life in France* by Julia Child and Alex Prud'homme. Surely those were more productive things to do than lie in bed for two hours and think crazy thoughts.

A wise and knowing friend told me weeks ago that no thoughts that anyone has at four in the morning are valid. They are always exaggerated and dramatic, whether or not the person has cancer or is hyped up on steroids, or just an insomniac. I think that's good advice.

Day 141

I chatted with my oncologist, Dr. K., about positive/negative attitudes and cancer, since there does seem to be a lot of talk about how one's attitude can affect the outcome of cancer.

"Well, no cancer patient ever gave themselves cancer by thinking bad thoughts, but stress and negativity do play a role in all disease and immune system function," he said.

"I have had patients with good attitudes die and negative patients who think they are about to die any day live another 20-40 years."

"Okay, that takes some of the pressure off of me having to have positive thoughts at all times!" I replied, relieved.

"If I had to pick one of my patients right now with the most positive attitude, who always has a smile or a joke or a funny comment, and who seems to be taking this whole journey in stride, it would be Amy Valentine, who comes to see him on Thursdays."

I'm sure he tells that to all his patients, but it made me feel good.

Day 142

My appetite has been gone since my last treatment. This morning I went downhill as the poison killed off the remaining healthy cells in my intestinal tract. Fortunately, my brother and neighbors were able to watch the kids while I took my meds and slept. I must be coming down off my steroid high because I'm a bit tired and depressed.

Everything feels heavy and hard and difficult today, and I know that's just a result of my sickly tummy and the strange cocktail of drugs in my system. I'm really a baby when it comes to ill health, even though I recognize that I'm pretty darn tough when it comes to all the needles and surgeries and nasty drugs I encounter on a weekly basis.

I just want to curl up on the sofa and have someone tell me everything is going to be okay. But the reality is, no one knows whether or not everything will be okay. If by okay, we mean a lifetime of 40 more years. So, do I want someone to lie to me just to make me feel good for a few minutes? Be a child again in a grown-up world? Or do I want to do this my hard realistic way — give me the facts, give me the truth, give me the strong medicine. Make me be a grown-up. I guess at 43, it's probably about time I grow up anyway. My mood shifts quickly these days depending on the variety of pharmaceuticals in my bloodstream and my personal conversations with God. For me that's good news, because I know the blues will pass and I'll be back in fighting spirit in a few minutes, a few hours, or perhaps this time, a few days.

Day 146

With Greg still in Brazil, I took the kids to San Antonio to see our former neighbors and celebrate their five-year-old's birthday. On the way, we made an emergency stop at a Starbuck's for a potty run and some food. Why do five-year-old boys suddenly need to go to the bathroom with dire urgency on a car trip, no matter how recently you've asked them if they need to go? According to several moms, this is a universal problem, and since I have relatively little knowledge of the inner workings of male plumbing, I will have to trust that the urge to pee somehow gets worked out as boys age. I don't remember any adult man suddenly and surprisingly needing to pee as if he had no idea that his bladder was filling up until it was about to explode. Since we had the aforementioned rapid dash to the bathroom, which of course was occupied, that meant the usual amount of dancing and prancing and complaining about the need to pee. We had a very loud entrance to Starbuck's.

I had my hat in the car, but usually walk around with my closely cropped hairstyle in daily life, so just went bald into the store. After about a half hour of the Valentine clan's energetic ordering, enthusiastic consuming, and many more trips from one side of Starbuck's to the other, we finally made our way out the door. As we were leaving, a nice looking 45-ish man, without a wedding band I might add, stopped me at the door. "Excuse me," he asked, "but is your shaved head a choice or a necessity?"

I was startled by the question but figured it was a bit of both. I told him, "it's a chemo-related hairstyle."

"I've had several family members go through cancer and I have several wigs left over if you need anything."

"Oh, I have several wigs at home. But it's so hot in the summer and my bald head is what it is so I just go bald or wear a sunhat most days."

We continued to chat for a bit. Then, this kind man I will probably never see again made my day by saying, "I think you're absolutely beautiful, and have such an amazing spirit about you. You are really an attractive woman."

And the women reading this will know what I'm talking about when he gave me that look that told me that he genuinely found me attractive. I was more stunned than anything so excused myself to get into my car with the kids.

Perhaps there are slim pickings for flirtations in New Braunfels, but this nice stranger I will never see again actually flirted with the crew-cut chemo mom with two kids at the Starbuck's. I will choose to think of the moment as my inner and outer beauty radiating and filling the Starbuck's with brightness and light. But maybe this guy just has a thing for bald heads and big fake boobs.

Day 151

Finished 3 of my 12 Taxol/Herceptin chemos. Now I have some strange post-chemo shaky thing going on. I'm sure I have a drug in my medicine chest of wonders to settle that, but I think I'm tired of drugs right now. Bad news is that my white blood cells were at 1700. At 1500 you can't get chemo. Since you need your weekly chemo to kill any possibly remaining cancer, you get a shot that's supposedly painful to boost white blood cell production. I had heard about this shot and thought you got it once, but no, today I found out that you get the shot daily for the duration of the chemo round. If the docs make the determination to give me the shot next week at Week 4, I will have 8 weeks of daily painful injections to add to my list of fun things to do in 2009.

I think I'm starting to see why folks just throw up their hands and go sit on a beach in Mexico trying some herbal remedy and sipping a margarita. Actually, I discovered pretty quickly why people go sit on a beach in Mexico but realized that's not my path.

I have remained relatively positive and sometimes even cheerful in the face of some awful surgeries, tests, weekly port lab draws, toxic poisons and steroid psychosis. But I think I'll take some Xanax and go hide under the sheets if I have to have 40 daily injections.

I saw a T-shirt the other day that read *Cancer messed with the wrong bitch*. Maybe I'll get that shirt and wear it to my next chemo. If I can't be strong on the inside, I can fake it on the outside. Bring it on, cancer, bring it on. Until that shirt arrives in the mail, I'll be the lump under the sheets in my bedroom.

Day 153

My cancer apparently comes with a side of Tourette's syndrome.

Thank goodness the steroids have calmed me down a bit and I have regained some mental control. I've never been given to cussing much. I like language and feel there are more powerful and meaningful words one can choose to express anger or fear or outrage.

Yet in the past four months, I've developed quite a potty mouth. In emails and in common conversation, the word cancer is inextricably linked to damned. I proudly wear my beautiful silver bracelet engraved with the words "Fuck Cancer", and just smile sweetly when people compliment it and ask if it might be from James Avery. It was a lovely gift from my dear friend Julie, who found it online. James Avery? No, I don't think so. And then I let them read the cursive engraving.

Because it's become acceptable in my mind to curse whenever I talk about cancer or chemo or surgery or drugs, the gateway is open to all sorts of four-letter words in everyday conversation. To my horror, I've caught myself cursing in front of small children, my minister, old ladies at the grocery store, acquaintances and even John our Mailman.

My friends and relatives put up with my sailor's dialect because they know the hell I'm going through. A few hells, shits, damns, and fucks aren't really going to make a difference one way or another, and if they help me let off a little steam, that's okay. I think the reality is that I've run out of words to express my cancer world. There are words for the pain from the surgeries, the awful side effects of the chemo, the insanity of the steroid psychosis. But I can't think of words bad enough to describe the fear of dying from a disease I can't control, can't explain, can't cure.

I can't explain my disbelief in a world where I can Skype my husband in Brazil and see his face blowing kisses at the kids through the computer, yet my oncologist can't tell me why I got cancer, if the treatment will help, or how to prevent it from returning.

I don't know how to prepare the people I love for the fact that I may not live my allotted 90 years and see my children grow up. Or I might. But I can't take it for granted like I did every day before March 27, 2009. Every day that I live, whether it's 1000 more days or 12,000 more, I will carry the word cancer someplace inside my mind.

After the initial shock and magnitude of my diagnosis wore off, I found moments that I didn't think about my disease. I have hours now that I don't obsess about my situation. It's harder right now when my very body reminds me of my illness from my bald head to my Frankenstein chest port and fake water balloon expander breasts.

Fastening my seat belt or putting my purse over my shoulder irritates my chest port, having the kids readjust when they lay their heads against my body to find a comfortable spot on my hard balloon breasts, lying down in my bed and having to cushion my body with a multitude of pillows ... all make my cancer world a bit inescapable.

But I have faith that one day my port will be out, and my treatment will be over, and my body will be returned to some semblance of the Amy I remember, I might have days that I forget about the word cancer. Maybe then my vocabulary won't need the expletive deletives to fill in the blanks for words that haven't been invented yet to describe the fear and pain and disbelief. Until then, you'll just have to fucking put up with me and my damned cancer.

Days 154 to 250

Yesterday when my tummy was out of control, one neighbor took my kids for most of the day while another fed them dinner and kept them busy until bedtime. Yet another neighbor called from the grocery store to see if she could pick up anything for me, and wanted to make sure I knew I could call her at any hour of the night since Greg was out of town. If there is a blessing in a diagnosis of cancer, it is the realization of how many people love and care for you and your family.

I've had friends from my past get back in touch with me and go out of their way to renew friendships, telling me how important I am in their lives even though we have allowed silence or distance to separate us. It doesn't surprise me that I know a lot of people — I'm an extrovert with outgoing children who also have a lot of friends, which doubles or triples the number of acquaintances I have. But, I have been surprised and touched by the kindness so many people have gone out of their way to show me.

I told a friend I was turning into a "kinder and gentler" Amy by my experience because I realize how only love and friendship matter in the long run. All the rest is just small potatoes. Maybe the rollercoaster isn't over this week, because as I write this, my eyes fill with tears, but they are tears of gratitude that by the grace of God, people love me to an extent that is in no way proportional to my worthiness.

Day 155

Now I understand the extreme fatigue that accompanies chemo. I'm lying on the sofa with my laptop next to me, too tired to walk across the room and answer the telephone or shut the front door that the kids have left open. So, the phone is ringing incessantly and we're air conditioning our 90-degree front porch. Kind friends offered to feed the kids and me dinner tonight but I'm not sure I can muster the energy to drive to their house. Maybe I just need a few cups of coffee, but somehow I don't think that would help. There are the steroid pills in my medicine chest but I dread possibly entering the world of steroid-induced psychosis. I'm more tired than I have ever felt in my life.

I wrote those previous sentences a few hours ago. Since then, my friends stepped up and helped me out in my time of great need: Sara is at a school friend's house and her mom offered to feed her dinner and get her ready for bed; Daniel is playing with another friend whose mom will drop him off right before we need to leave to go to dinner.

With only one child to take to dinner and three hours to rest, I think I'll make it through the day. How do people do it without the hordes of help I have? I chatted with a woman at chemo two weeks ago who was there with a friend. She said the cancer patient was a single mom with a quadriplegic son and didn't have good health insurance so the breast cancer diagnosis was a huge financial burden. It doesn't matter if she's at Stage 1 or Stage 3, she is walking a rougher path than I am. I'm going to go take a nap now.

Day 156

Two weeks ago when I was receiving my infusion of Taxol and Herceptin, Greg was out of town. I was also still on my heavy doses of steroids so suffered from steroid-induced mania. All of this resulted in a ghoulishly funny conversation. While leaving the oncology office, I called Greg .

"Greg, guess what happened at chemo today. Two seats over from mine, a woman had an allergic reaction to Herceptin," I said.

"What happened? That could happen to you still, right?"

"Well, there was a flurry of activity with nurses pushing drugs into the IV and the doctors came over from the other side of the oncology building," I continued.

"What did the woman look like when it was happening?" Greg asked.

"I couldn't see her very well. She just looked asleep to me. She was covered up with blankets."

"They covered her up? Covered her up with the blanket?"

"Yes, covered her with the blanket."

"OMG! That's not a good sign when they pull the blanket over your head! She was dead?"

I laughed hysterically due to the steroids at the miscommunication, "No, no, no. She was covered up to her neck in blankets as if she were cold, that's all! She was still alive!"

The only way I knew it was a Herceptin allergic reaction was because my nurse told me in a round-about sort of way. I asked her what was happening and she said quietly, "Oh, I can't talk about it. But, I'm glad you didn't have an allergic reaction to the Herceptin."

Day 157

First, Happy 42nd Birthday Greg! Second, I fear I am turning into a 17 year old boy. I look at breasts all the time! Because I get brand new breasts soon, I observe different sizes, various shapes, how women's breasts look under clothes, in bathing suits. It's like shopping for a new car.

You never see the Highlander Hybrids on the road until you are shopping for cars. Then you see them everywhere. They park next to you at the grocery store, pull up behind you at red lights, and pass you on the freeway.

It's the same way with breasts, although I have an even better chance to see breasts than car models because boobs are everywhere. Being a mom, opportunities abound for seeing a wide variety of boobs on a daily basis — women with babies nurse around me, I go into women's changing rooms where women undress, and I have friends who are kind enough to let me see and feel their breasts. What, women go around feeling each other's breasts?

Not usually, but since my diagnosis of breast cancer, not only have I been felt up by more people than ever before in 43 years, but I have had the opportunity to feel other women's breasts, which I had never done before. It seems crazy, but it's actually been quite helpful as I try to decide on the exact size I'd like to be once my expanders have been removed and the gummy bear silicone gel implants are in place. I have also discovered which of my friends have had augmentation. Many of my friends have killer bust lines (not as dangerous as mine were, however), but I had no idea that several of them had been artificially enhanced.

One especially generous and kind friend let me see and feel her breasts and discussed various details such as implant and bra sizes. She looks fabulous by the way, so while I've never been a fan of the augmented look, the new gummy bear silicone gel implants are so wonderful, I now recommend them to anyone wanting a perkier décolletage.

After much shopping around and making observations about my friends' various cleavage sizes and bras, I decided to upgrade a size or so. Of course, I had to let my plastic surgeon decide if my body could handle two more ounces on each side. Dr. H was more than happy to increase my bust line and joked that a few more ounces was not going to change my career, as I always told him I didn't want "stripper boobs."

Day 162

While I fancy no return trip to steroid-psychosis land, I have voluntarily put myself back on my crazy drugs. I chatted with some physician friends and my infusion nurse over the weekend and decided there couldn't be much harm in dosing myself with my leftover steroid pills to try to raise my white blood cell counts.

No one thinks it's going to do much good, but it might. They all made me promise that Greg would be allowed to tell me I was manic and needed to stop the steroids.

I found that last part very funny. Of course if Greg tells me I'm crazy and need to stop the drugs, I will. He's my steady rock in these stormy waters.

So, for the three days leading up to my next chemo, I'm taking the Decadron pills. Maybe this time, I'll clean out the closets and power wash the French doors leading to the backyard. If I seem a little more wacky than usual, blame the drugs.

Day 163

Greg and I had our first real fight since my cancer diagnosis. It was bound to happen. After all, the honeymoon only lasts so long. For four months, I've been especially meek and full of love and kindness, when I'm not a raging crazy woman making cancer my bitch.

So, last night, I'm exhausted after a full day of Sunday school, church, a trip to the Apple store, and swimming at my friend Julie's pool. I haven't slow down much since cancer came to call — if anything, I ramp up the activities because I don't want to have my children miss anything remotely educational or fun.

The kids were excited about the church's ice cream social that night, and I had hoped Greg would take pity on my fatigue and take the kids. He said he would after he ran into the shower, but I just wasn't in the mood to wait.

When he wasn't forthcoming about stepping in to help and wasn't planning to go himself until later, I was grumpy and cranky. Greg poked the bear by accusing me of acting passive aggressive, and wanted me to just come out and say what was bothering me. I'm not usually called "passive aggressive;" I'm aggressive aggressive if anything!

I angrily said, "I have cancer. I wanted you to take the kids to the ice cream social so I could go to sleep!"

Greg replied, "If you're going to use cancer as part of an argument every time something bothers you, I should just stop now because why even try to argue?"

After realizing how wrong I was and how right he was, (a few hours later) I started laughing.

I kissed my husband and apologized, saying "you know, I'm going to be 90, still using cancer as a reason to get you to do things for me..."Greg, go get my walker please. I had cancer back in 2009..."

Day 164

Today, I called my oncologist's nurse, "I need a prescription for medical marijuana. Can you ask Dr. K about that?"

"Are you having nausea?" the kind nurse asked.

"Not so much. I wanted to make sure I took advantage of all the opportunities this nifty cancer diagnosis afforded me."

She laughed, "Oh, I don't think medical marijuana is legal in the state of Texas, but I can't wait to ask Dr. K."

"Make sure to tell him I need the prescription by this Friday coz there's a party...oh, and I'm suddenly having chemo-related nausea."

When the nurse called me back, she said that Dr. K told me he could write the prescription but I'd have to fill it in California and move the party to that state.

"Are you having nausea because we have other medication we can prescribe," she said.

"No, no, if I can't get the medical marijuana, I'll be fine."

She then said I had made their day in the office with my marijuana request and was completely crazy.

I replied, "oh, you say that to all your patients."

The nurse said, "well, you're crazier than most."

Greg does have a lot of frequent flier miles...hmmm... party in San Francisco next weekend anyone?

Day 166

Yesterday my ring finger on my right hand had a small blister that looked like an ant bite. I was trying to figure out if a bug had bitten me until I woke up this morning with two on the same finger and three small red blisters on my pinkie finger. My mom encouraged me to call the oncologist on call to see if this was a chemo-related side effect. Sure enough, I have Taxol/Taxatere related extremity blisters. The doctor sympathized with me but told me there wasn't a lot I could do, and since the hands have so many nerve endings, I was probably in for a painful weekend. He said not to bandage them, and suggested I could spread baby teething cream (really?) on them to numb the pain if necessary. At Daniel's soccer game this morning, I watched small red dots pop out on the palms of both hands and small blisters start to form on my left hand fingers as well. Fortunately, the only ones that hurt were the original three or four on my right hand. I immediately began taking my supplements for neuropathy and am hoped for the best. The doc on call did say that Dr. K may delay my next treatment by a week to allow my hands to heal.

I don't want that so said, "I'm sure it will be much better by Thursday. In fact, my fingers feel better already." So how does a mom do her job without using her hands? Did you ever try to put soccer shin guards, socks and soccer cleats on a squirming five-year-old boy without using the pads of your fingers? I'm quite talented, obviously.

Day 167

This weekend I spent most of it in bed under the covers, hiding from the realities of my cancer world. The painful blisters continued to hurt and I felt completely helpless to do much about them. Without the use of my fingers, staying in bed seemed like the best plan. After taking my supplements, and dredging my hands in a special salve a friend gave me, the blisters seem better this afternoon. I'm a bit fearful that this does not bode well for the next five weeks, since the blisters are caused by a toxic buildup of the poisons. The body is smart and protects the vital organs by pushing the toxins to the extremities. So far my toes are fine, but with my luck and my current negative attitude, I'm expecting red welts on them any minute. Greg assures me that he has confidence I will rally. Maybe even by tonight.

Day 168

Cancer can't keep me down for long. I rallied as my husband predicted, and am back to my somewhat cheery self. It helps that the blisters seem better today. None of the have actually broken through the skin, and appear as tender swollen welts on a few places on my fingers and palms. They feel like tiny irritated splinters on several points on my hands that especially hurt when I pick something up or rub against something on that part of my skin. It hurt to hold my son's hand yesterday, but to-day the pain and swelling have subsided. So, I'm taking advantage of the reprieve and holding both my children's hands as much as possible.

Day 171

Since the doctors can't tell me much about my cancer — why I got it, if I'll get more cancer, what I can do to prevent recurrence — I spend a lot of time second-guess-ing the past choices in my life. Some of them are silly — what if I had only fabric shower curtains for the 20 years preceding my diagnosis? Some of them are profound — what if I had married my college sweetheart and had my children before the age of 30? I expected my oncologist to ask me for a list of personal care products, places lived, bags of Cheetos consumed, number of airline miles accrued when I was first diagnosed. But no, other than finding out what my occupation had been and what my family cancer history was, there was no interest shown in Oil of Olay moisturizer or pesticides on thin-skinned peaches. The doctor never even asked me about birth control pills, which would seem an obvious breast cancer risk to the casual observer, yet it never shows up in breast cancer risk questionnaires. What if my cancer was caused by my lifetime addiction to Crest toothpaste? I have brushed regularly with the same brand of toothpaste at least twice a day for the past 30 years. Couldn't that have had an impact on my illness? It's nice to have no cavities, but wouldn't I rather have fillings and no cancer?

What if switching toothpaste was all it required to live another healthy 50 years? There is a lot of talk about antiperspirant and deodorant use contributing to various cancers, especially breast and lymph node cancers. So, for a few weeks I diligently gave up my beloved Dove Ultimate Cool Essentials antiperspirant for some quirky all natural deodorant. I finally realized I was stinky and would rather be fresh even if it took years off my life. What a conclusion. At the time it seemed quite deep but now makes me chuckle. I'm sure if I knew that Dove Ultimate Cool Essentials contributed to my cancer, I would happily substitute another brand, even one that did not make me feel as fresh as a daisy, but without definitive proof, I'm reluctant to make the switch.

Should Greg and I have bought a new home in an Austin suburb as we planned a few years ago and avoided the ancient Indian burial ground our current house is built on? What if I would have moved to France after college when I was still slightly fluent and spent years eating and drinking European food and beverages? Was my fertile nature getting pregnant quickly in my mid-30s a harbinger of the estrogen-driven tumors my body would later produce? Should I have been more wary of the future illness that would drastically change my life, my attitude and to some extent my personality? Friends have suggested changing my diet and lifestyle and I replied, "Then I'd better stop eating lots of fruits and veggies and start drinking and smoking heavily since the low-fat, high fruit and veggie diet I had before didn't work very well."

I had a McDonald's cheeseburger once in a while and could stand to go to the gym more often like everyone else, but my pre-cancer lifestyle was pretty healthy. So I continue to wonder about my past and worry about the future.

A very level-headed friend heard about my general discontent and described it as having a "change the channel" moment. She said she periodically will think life is like a TV and all she has to do is change the channel to find her "other, better life." I thought that described my unhappiness perfectly. But I'm not very unhappy, it's just a low-level irritation in wanting to escape my real world by daydreaming about an alternate universe.

In fact, since my diagnosis, I'm actually happier in general, because I don't sweat the small stuff. Major issues such as death and surgery and pain depress me, but I live each day appreciating the wheat and ignoring the chaff. Ultimately, when I daydream about another life a different Amy would have chosen, my heart comes back to the same place. Perhaps that Amy wouldn't have breast cancer at age 42, but she also wouldn't know Greg or Sara or Daniel. All my friends and in-laws and neighbors would be different. The hands that reach out to me when I'm sad would be different hands. The kind souls who hold me in their prayers when I'm low would have different faces. The people who call or text or email just to tell me they are thinking about me wouldn't be the ones I know now. So, my heart answers my philosophical life musings by telling me I would rather have my life cut short by cancer, if that is indeed my fate, and experience the love I know now than live to 90 on a different channel.

Day 180

I'm at the top of the mountain, beginning my downhill trip as my darling German neighbor commented, on my halfway mark to this round of chemo. Seven of my 12

Taxol/Herceptin infusions behind me now... whew. It seems like it's been an arduous uphill climb and I'm looking forward to the easy ride down. (That is a joke because I don't think there is such an animal in Cancer World.) My white blood cell counts were the highest yet at 1800 (yippee!) which caused my iPhone to bing off the wall as I sent out informative texts to my friends and received happy messages back.

So, I avoided the dreaded shots one more week. Dr. K told me I looked and seemed great — good spirits, good color, healthy attitude and sense of humor intact. He compared this to the last few weeks when I've been a little down in the dumps. Really, is it unusual for someone who has cancer to be a bit blue? I would think it more unusual for someone with cancer to be perky and upbeat.

I think Dr. K is right about my attitude improving, because I'm starting to notice funny little moments that make me laugh.

Two days ago at the grocery store, I had on my hat but no wig. At the checkout counter, the teenage clerk tried to sell me shampoo and conditioner that was the HEB special for the day. When I commented in a matter-of-fact tone, "no thanks, I don't have hair," and took off my hat, I expected to get a smile or funny comment from the clerk. Instead, he just kept on checking my groceries and making small talk as if it were the most ordinary thing for someone to come through his line without hair. His reaction to my attempt at humor amused me to no end. And I do continue to wash my peach fuzz head in the shower with whatever shampoo I had last spring when I had hair. I was reading the label this morning and realized it was the "anti-flat, volume boosting" formula. Again, I had to laugh. But, if anyone needs volume-boosting shampoo, it would be me!

Day 187

I'm off to my 8th round of Taxol/Herceptin infusions today and had the hardest time sleeping last night and getting up this morning. More dreams about houses. Really, this has to stop. I have had at least twenty dreams involving houses. I wake up exhausted from all the real estate shopping. Someone told me that the house represents the body in dream language. Well, there's definitely a lot of changes going on in my "house" if that's what's prompting my dreams.

I dread today's appointment, mainly because there are so many uncertainties about my side effects, symptoms and treatments. My right armpit has been hurting, but it's hard to say if it's inflammation from my breast expander or a swollen lymph node.

Greg assures me that it can't be that the cancer has spread further into my body because when I actually had a breast cancer lump and lymph node involvement, none of it hurt. It's more likely I have an infection or cut or something on my hand, causing my lymph nodes to act up. If it's even a lymph node.

There has been so much trauma to my breasts, under-arms and lymph system through surgery, it's hard to say what exactly is going on. Maybe my five-year-old who likes to pull on my arms when he's holding my hand has just irritated that area. But it all combines to make me es-pecially dread today's appointment.

Thank God for Xanax and good friends. If I start cry-ing in the oncologist's office, where I'm known for my cheery demeanor and irreverent attitude, I'll have my trusty drug and a shoulder to lean on. Since I pre-medi-cated myself a while ago, I'm about to fall asleep and still have to make Daniel's lunch, put Emler numbing cream on my port, and get him off to preschool. Today just seems hard, but no one promised me it would be easy...

Day 188

Well, I made it through another round of Taxol/Her-ceptin chemo! My counts were 1500, barely squeaking by without the dreaded shots to boost my white blood cells. My other worries wound up as minor concerns in Cancer World. The oncology nurse practitioner examined my sore underarm and determined it was caused by my water balloon expander pack. The blisters on my fingers are not a common side effect of the Taxol. Again, not a cause for worry. Lisa, the nurse practitioner, said it might be more of an allergic reaction than anything else. I went ahead with treatment, and should treat any subsequent blisters with over-the-counter Benadryl or Zyrtec. I can also ice my hands during future Taxol treatments to slow down circulation and prevent the Taxol from reaching the fingertips. Since I already have poor circulation and perennially frigid fingers, that doesn't sound like much fun. Lisa didn't even want to change the mix of steroids/Benadryl in my drip. If I get more blisters this round, they may add some of the steroids to my subsequent drips, but everyone would like to avoid the steroid psychosis I encountered last time. Was I more obviously crazy than I thought if the oncology office is scared to add steroids to my mix even when I had painful welts?

It has been interesting that for each round of Taxol/Herceptin, I've presented different side effects each week. I wonder what's in store for me this time? Several of my girlfriends have told me that breast cancer runs in their families and they just assume my fate will be their future. This is so hard both physically and mentally that I cringe when I hear that and pray that no one I know will ever have to take this journey.

I think it's helpful that they are prepared for a cancer diagnosis and treatment if it strikes them, but know that no one can understand how awful this is until you have to walk the walk. Maybe I'm just weaker than most because I'm counting down the days at this point, dreading each treatment, side effect and symptom. I cling to the adage that what doesn't kill me makes me stronger. After four more weeks of hell, I should be so strong that nothing will knock me down. Bring it on, cancer. Bring it on.

Day 189

How many posts have had this title? I feel like a truck hit me this morning. I'm so tired and everything hurts, mentally more than physically. It all seems so hard and so long and so difficult. My muscles ache, my stomach hurts, my intestines are screwed up, everything burns, my hands are puffy and starting to get welts, plus the extreme fatigue is crazy. I have other symptoms I can't even talk about, and heaven knows I reveal all in this blog so you have to use your imagination! I see my acupuncturist in an hour and then am taking a Xanax and sleeping and maybe I'll dream about that other life without cancer. I can't believe I have 27 more days walking through this particular chemo drug hell. What's the song about when you go through hell, just keep on walking and maybe the devil won't know you're there? I think the devil spotted me a couple of months ago ...

Day 194

Thank you to my new friend Amy M. who invited me to attend the Breast Cancer Resource Center's Annual Champagne Brunch Gala and Fundraiser today. Amy is a two-time breast cancer survivor who spotted me at Hill Elementary and came over to welcome me to the Cancer Club. My bald head in morning assembly gave me away, I guess. Today it was nice to see 500 breast cancer patients, survivors and supporters acting like any other roomful of horny women when hunky firemen stood onstage and stripped in support of breast cancer research. Maybe you had to be there to fully understand the connection between beefy firefighters and breast cancer. I wasn't complaining. I wouldn't have been so reluctant to join the Cancer Club if I had known my membership came with hot, half-naked firefighters.

I surprised myself a bit by wavering between wearing a wig or not to this event. In everyday life, I have no problem popping a hat on my patchy crew cut and running around town. It is what it is, after all. But, whenever Greg and I go out to dinner or I get dressed up in any way (except for church where I figure God understands the bald look), I tend to wear a wig. Amy M. said she had never worn a wig except when her Kindergartener asked her to, so that encouraged me to go bald. I figured a BCRC event was the one truly acceptable place to go wigless, because it was a cancer support function after all. When we got there, I was surprised to see that I was one of only a handful of bald women. There were wigs in abundance (I'm an expert wig spotter now) and lots of scarves and turbans. The ebullient woman next to me immediately asked me about the wig choice and said she was such a private person that she chose to wear a wig throughout her cancer treatment. I guess I'm the opposite, because my life is fairly transparent. Anyone who has a public blog where she discusses the Brazilian effects of chemotherapy can't really claim to be much of a private person.

Of course, one of my more perceptive, introverted friends once drunkenly commented about my transparency; that there is no better person to hide the secrets of their soul than an extreme extrovert like me. By choosing to show all to the world, everyone assumes what they see is what they get. So, the choice is really mine to reveal exactly and precisely what I want when I want and how I want it. That sounds pretty complicated to me, but I tend not to argue with drunken girlfriends who know too many deep secrets about me anyway.

Today my side effects are minimal, or maybe it was the extrovert in me enjoying the energy of the crowd and my new friend that pepped me up. My main complaint is a twitchy right eye. Seriously, I have this nerve twitch that is driving me crazy and probably not related to chemo or cancer at all, unless it's the dreaded breast cancer of the eyeball. Maybe I just exhausted my eyelid from all the ogling of firefighters. I guess given the champagne gala, speaker Rue McClanahan's naughty speech about the joys of growing older (she is on her sixth husband), and the half-naked firefighters, it was a pretty good day.

Day 195

Today is starting out pretty well. I'm feeling fine and not extremely tired. My fingers started hurting last night, and I dreaded waking up with red welts again. But, no. Two fingers have the start of my little ant bite marks, but they aren't getting worse. I'm not complaining, but it's a bit schizophrenic with my good day/bad day chemo effects. I never know which side of the bed I'm waking up on. I guess as long as I keep waking up, I'll take the bad with the good. And the good with the bad!

Day 196

"If I had known how much work it was going to be, I never would have gotten cancer," I complained to my oncologist.

Today I saw a dermatologist because I have an inflamed sebaceous cyst in my lower back region. I had to get prior permission from my oncologist to have a dermatologist excise the cyst or give it a shot of steroids.

Since I'm currently bald, I had the doctor do a mole check too. I've discovered beauty marks in places I never knew I had them. For example: the top of my scalp and soles of my feet! Geez, get your minds out of the gutter.

The dermatologist looked at the cyst and then told me, "you're not going to like what I am about to tell you."

My heart plummeted, as someone who has had a cancer diagnosis can understand.

"Is it cancer?" I hesitantly asked.

"Oh no, not cancer," she says. "I can't take off the cyst today so you'll have to see a surgeon."

Really? Shame on you for scaring me like that!

"Should I see a general surgeon or a plastic surgeon, since I have both on speed dial," I asked.

"I don't usually refer patients to a plastic surgeon for cyst or mole removal that's not the on the face," she said. "The buttocks area is not considered a cosmetic area."

I shot back, "Don't tell my husband that! He would be quite upset if *that* part of my body was disfigured."

I called to see if my plastic surgeon Dr. H can just take care of the back cyst, flip me over and then finish my boobs. No, it can't be that easy. Dr. H doesn't operate on these cysts and in fact can't do the reconstruction surgery until I first take care of the cyst. He couldn't operate if I have *any* sort of infection.

Even though the dermatologist prescribed a month's worth of antibiotics to clear up any infection, I still have to see my general surgeon to determine a plan. But I can't simply take the drugs as prescribed. I have to call my oncologist first to get approval to take the medicine. The oncology nurse reminds me that I can't have any surgery in October while I'm on Taxol in case my white blood cell count is low. Sigh. It's so complicated.

So, I have an appointment with my general surgeon for next week to have him examine this troublesome cyst. Worst case scenario is that I have general surgery in November to remove the cyst when my white blood cell counts increase. Then, my boob surgery will be pushed back to December.

I was thinking while all this phone calling and rescheduling and planning was going on that a year ago the thought of possibly having general surgery to remove a cyst near my spine would have freaked me out. Now, it's small potatoes. I'm relieved that it's not cancer. For someone who had never had general anesthesia before last April, I now have three or possibly four surgeries on my plate in the next year. All of my clever friends who have been teasing me about a bountiful Thanksgiving when I give gratitude for my new cleavage may have to think of clever jokes around a Christmas season theme instead.

Day 202

Yesterday, I told Greg my "soles hurt" and he hugged me. I realized he misunderstood and thought I said "my soul's hurt." Neuropathy, fatigue and some intestinal discomfort/nausea have been my main side effects this go round. Along with my fingers being tingly and slightly numb, yesterday my feet were starting to hurt. After my funny homophone mix-up with Greg, I repeated my Freudian slip to a girlfriend on the phone, and got a similar sympathetic reaction. Neither my husband nor my girlfriend seemed to think it odd that I would say, "My soul is hurt." I would consider that a very unusual and quirky thing for someone to say, even someone with cancer. Perhaps my soul is hurt.

Perhaps these people who love me recognize the depth of my pain and think it a perfectly normal thing for me to acknowledge. In Sunday School this morning, our class discussed the rock band U2 and lead singer Bono's spirituality. Bono was quoted as saying something about "lament being the outcry of the overwhelmed." Lament is a lovely old-fashioned word that always seemed to have a bit of a whiny connotation before cancer came to call.

Now, I think what I describe as my anger at God isn't really anger. It's a lament. My discussions with God have always been more of an incredulous, "really, God, this is my path? Bilateral breast cancer at 42? Flan-like paste during CT scans every three months for the rest of my life? Having to explain to my five-year-old that my cancer isn't like Grandpa Jerry's metastatic lung cancer that killed him two years ago? I'm crying out to God when I'm overwhelmed. And most days, I'm overwhelmed.

Day 203

Last night a friend asked how my mastectomy scars were healing. I told her they were fine, but I realized that even after my reconstruction surgery, I probably wasn't going to ever look that good naked again.

She chuckled and replied, "You know, I'm not either."

She continued, "We're not 25 anymore, and what does it matter? Greg loves you and is happy you're alive regardless of what your body and scars look like. Neither of us was ever a playboy bunny or swimsuit model after all."

I guess Cancer doesn't have much to do with Time's effects anyway.

Today, I went to my general surgeon to have him examine my lower back/buttock cyst to see if I needed surgery to remove it. It's just a sebaceous cyst so he could numb it and take it off in the office.

I also found out that when he removes my port next summer, that will be an outpatient office procedure. I find it odd that the surgeon can remove a shunt into my heart in an office procedure when inserting it required general anesthesia and a hospital visit.

After the procedure was over, he asked if he could see my reconstructed breasts. Hmmm…that sounded creepy when I wrote it. It really wasn't since he was the doctor who performed my mastectomy after all. And my mother-in-law and a nurse were both present.

Dr. M immediately praised my plastic surgeon and said he's seen enhancements that didn't look as good as my breasts now. And this is before the final reconstruction. Maybe I might look pretty good naked after my reconstruction. And with my new enhanced figure, perhaps swimsuit model isn't such a stretch…

Day 206

For the first time in months, I drove through Wendy's and had fast food for lunch. I've been paranoid about everything I put in my mouth since March 27th. I never thought I ate a lot of fast food, but when I ordered, the words "Number one combo with cheese, no onion, extra pickles please" rolled off my tongue.

Perhaps I was a bit too familiar with Wendy's cheeseburgers. When the clerk handed me my burger, salad and iced tea, she said the usual Wendy's phrase, "See you tomorrow."

I almost burst into laughter.

See you tomorrow. What a positively lovely thing to say.

It's like the surgeon who discharged me from the hospital after my double mastectomy. When I made a comment about wanting 16 years to see both kids through college, the surgeon said, "why not 40 years, 50 years?" Who knew surgeons and cheeseburgers came with a side of hope?

Day 209

I've sat with an idea of how cancer changes the survivor that has come to me over the past few months in dribs and drabs. I was unwilling or unable to acknowledge it until last week.

The therapist and cancer survivor who ran the parent support group I attended in the past sent me an email and succinctly put this interesting concept into words. Her sentence struck me and resonated throughout that day and that night and the next day and ever since.

"From the outside looking in it may appear our lives return to "normal", but we will be forever changed, and not necessarily for the worst."

Could it be that my experience with cancer might change me in a way that is "not necessarily for the worst?"

Day 212

One of my closest friends gave birth today to her fourth baby. Welcome Vivi! While the birth of a new baby is always a source of joy, this birth has a special significance to me. Julie's due date was October 22nd, which is the date of my last hard chemo round. Back in March, when I was first diagnosed, Julie had recently found out she was pregnant. When we counted up the weeks of my chemo and her pregnancy, we realized we would both be walking uncomfortable paths at the same time. While neither of us compared cancer to pregnancy, many of the side effects and experiences of the subsequent six months would be quite similar. When I was suffering the worst of my chemo-brain, Julie was having pregnancy-brain. Several times one of us would call the other and completely blank on why we had originally picked up the phone. Julie laughed that between us, we had one complete brain!

When I was in the weeks of my steroid psychosis, my hormonal friend empathized with my insomnia and racing emotions. Last week, Julie's obstetrician put her on steroids to increase her platelet count to allow her to have an epidural during labor. So, it became my turn to sympathize with her craziness.

When I complained about physical discomfort with my chest port and expander balloon breasts, let alone the myriad other chemo-related horrors, Julie would have similar pregnancy-related discomforts. Her giant belly prevented her from sleeping in certain positions, and the indigestion and nausea that accompanies many pregnancies mimicked my own discomfort.

So, today while I'm having trouble typing and holding various items due to my neuropathy, I cheer for the fact that Julie's week-early delivery signals the imminent end of my chemo. Months after my cancer diagnosis, I realized that Julie called me every single day, often just leaving a message. When I asked her later about that, she told me she deliberately called me each day and some days were hard for her to call because she didn't know what to say, how to empathize with me, how to help me through such a hard experience. What a gift, my dear friend.

In the midst of my illness tinged with its undeniable mortality issues, I celebrate the birth of new life. Is there anything more helpless and frail than a newborn baby? And at the same time is there anything that shouts louder the strength and determination of the human nature than the miracle of labor, delivery and new life? Helpless, frail, strong and determined. Any wonder I see similarities and rejoice at this day?

Day 215

With October being Breast Cancer Awareness Month, my cancer and I are quite the trend. At my local grocery store, instead of ignoring my crew cut, clerks smile proudly and ask if I have breast cancer. It's like showing off a new baby. Everyone talks about Breast Cancer Awareness Month and wears their pink ribbons and supportive T-shirts, but actually meeting someone who has breast cancer delights the public and deems me a rock star.

I'm happy to discuss my illness and treatment with anyone, but am still a bit surprised when everyone from the 17-year-old high school boy to the 50-year-old store manager all begin casual conversations about what used to be an awkward topic.

This month, the grocery clerks ask all shoppers to consider making a donation to a local breast cancer support organization. I get a pass for already donating to the cause, willing or not!

When I insist on making a donation, the clerk inadvertently pressures all other shoppers in my line to also make a donation by loudly discussing my disease, treatment and symptoms. Even though it's usually cold in grocery stores and I almost always wear a hat, I now automatically take off the hat in my shopping line, prepared for the overt sale.

I wear my T-shirts "Yes, they're fake. My real ones tried to kill me," and "Cancer, you messed with the wrong bitch!" proudly this month and see pink ribbons everywhere.

Football players have pink ribbons on their helmets during games, giant helium pink ribbon balloons adorn retail stores, and window displays in stores all over town announce the cause. Not that I wanted to join this club, but you know the drama-queen in me loves the attention.

If I had to get cancer, at least I got the trendy kind. I wonder if men get the same attention during Prostate Cancer Month? Can you imagine every bald man getting asked if he has prostate cancer?

Day 218

A friend of mine in New York City sent me an email telling me it was so good that I had Greg and the kids, because I had no choice but to fight and get better. I thought that was beautifully phrased. No choice. And my family has no choice but to fight with me.

That's not such a blessing for them. As much as I would like to protect my loved ones from the battle, my transparent nature means my friends and family get it all.

When I see how my journey affects Sara and Daniel, my heart aches not knowing if they suffer or benefit from seeing me at my best and my worst, because believe me, my children have witnessed both extremes.

I try to cry only when in the shower or late at night when the kids are asleep, but every so often a TV commercial or card or email will surprise me and the tears will start to flow.

Have you seen the insurance company ad with the little girl asking to borrow her dad's car and then suddenly she turns into an 18-year-old and runs out the door? To parents, our children will always be the helpless little sweet tots we had to take care of, even when they grow up.

At Sara's back-to-school night when Greg and I were looking through Sara's daily writing journal, Greg pointed out the entry, "Mom has brest cancr. It maks me sad."

One day Daniel's preschool teachers told me about Daniel's art projects. He was playing with play-doh and announced, "I've made a breast cancer ribbon!" And sure enough he had.

While driving in the car with both kids a few weeks ago, Daniel had a stuffed sea turtle with him. He was telling Sara something about his turtle helping people with cancer, or that the turtle had cancer. So, I stopped being a passive sponge soaking up the kids' conversation, and asked what the turtle did. Daniel said the turtle helps breast cancer. I tried to make sense of that and said, "You mean the turtle helps people who have breast cancer?"

Daniel laughed and clarified, "No, Mommy, the turtle helps other TURTLES with breast cancer!" Of course!

Do other parents have these conversations with their children? I'd rather go back to discussing how we would make rocket booster shoes that fly or where the water goes when it drains out of the bathtub.

Next week the kids are going down to the Child Development lab at the University of Texas to complete a study for 3, 5 and 7-year-olds about their understanding of invisible things. The researcher was explaining that some of the concepts will be invisible objects such as germs and imaginary friends.

I asked if God, dead relatives, angels or cancer cells will be discussed. The Valentine children are well-versed on those invisible concepts. They have no choice.

Day 236

Tonight while watching Sara at Tae Kwon Do, I had one of the most profound conversations about cancer ... with a 10-year-old.

This young girl saw my crew cut and flat out asked, "did you have cancer?"

I was so impressed with her proper use of verb tense (past) that my heart immediately warmed to her. "Yes, I did, but I'm better now."

To which she replied, "a friend of mine had cancer, twice, but she's all better now too."

Immediately, my cancer somehow seemed less important to me in the light of a 10-year-old with cancer. I asked about her friend and if she had lost her hair. I mentioned that when kids get cancer they almost always get better, because their bodies are growing and changing so fast that they respond well to the medicine.

We had a lovely, honest conversation. This little girl even asked what kind of cancer I'd had. I expected questions about my breasts, but kept my end of the conversation purely PG. Ten-year-old girls don't need to know about mastectomies.

Then she added the words that touched me deeply, "my friend's okay now, and I'm sure you'll be fine too."

Deep in the heart of my darkness four months ago, the broken child in me just wanted to hear, "everything is going to be okay." I could have heard that sentence every hour of every day from March 27th on. It still sounds pretty good to me seven months later, and today I'm considerably healthier and saner.

No one volunteers those words to a cancer patient, because the truth is that no one knows everything will be okay. I would have to ask Greg, friends, family just to tell me everything would be okay. The words were strangely comforting, even when I was the one writing the script.

And this sweet little girl blessed me with her innocent confidence. "I'm sure you'll be fine too."

Day 239

Today was my Herceptin infusion day since that "more gentle" chemo drug continues for a full year. I was surprisingly anxious, even though this particular drug doesn't cause me any noticeable side effects. What it's doing to my heart however remains to be seen, take that phrase as you will.

On a physical level, all of my past echocardiograms have been normal. On a deeper level, my cardiologist wouldn't be able to see those changes.

I think I dreaded returning to the scene of the crime where the memories live of the Amy who was ill and made more sick by nasty poisons. Since it had been three weeks, I was delighted to visit with my oncologist again. I had brought homemade cookies along with my Christmas card and bluntly thanked him for "saving my life".

He might have been taken aback by gratitude on such a grand scale, but recovered and answered, "all in a day's work," which is probably true for a physician in his field.

He examined me and admired my new soft breasts (in a professional manner of course). When he returned after I dressed, he told me how great and healthy I looked. And then, to my surprise, his eyes became misty and he smiled affectionately as if I were one of his daughters, and said, "You are just so full of life".

I would think an oncologist would cease to be touched by the resilience of a cancer patient since every day all his patients are walking the same walk. As much as I would like to think I exhibit unusual strength and grace, the reality is that I have joined a club of amazing men and women who fight with courage and grace.

Could it be that in cancer's attempt to steal my life, the battle to save it gave me more life than before?

Day 250

At chemo a few months ago, a patient across from me was complaining about neuropathy in her extremities from the Taxol. We began chatting about the various supplements you can take to help prevent nerve tingling and numbness. I asked her if she had breast cancer and she replied, "ovarian."

I immediately thought how glad I was that I wasn't in her shoes because of the low survival rate of those diagnosed with ovarian cancer.

After hearing that I had small children at home with me, she said, "oh my, at least my baby is 26 years old".

Shockingly, she was thinking the same thing: "I'm so glad I'm not in this woman's shoes." Perhaps our trials are meted out according to our endurance, because I wouldn't trade my situation for hers, nor I suspect, would she trade hers for mine.

How can I not be affected by the mortality evidenced by that simple conversation? In four months since diagnosis, I felt profoundly different. While I joked about my big boobs and bald head, it was really the internal transformation that would carry me through this cancer world and out onto the other side.

Every conversation seemed imbued with a deeper meaning, relationships were intensified, and emotions were heightened. If I barely recognize the external Amy I saw in the mirror, I would be more baffled by the person on the inside. Who would I be in another year? In another ten? The Taxol may cause numbness in my fingers and toes, but the cancer experience seemed to have had the reverse effect on my heart.

Who would I be internally and externally after the exhaustive and revolutionary changes my body and soul would endure?

Eight months after diagnosis, I had completed my initial mastectomy, most of my reconstruction expander saline fills, three months of "hard" chemo, and three months of Taxol and Herceptin. I still had another nine months of Herceptin chemo, reconstructive surgery, and 38 daily rounds of radiation.

In addition, my oncologist would recommend monthly shots in the stomach for three years to absorb any extra estrogen to more fully protect me from a future recurrence of cancer. Daily Tamoxifen pills would continue for ten years. These adventures continue in my second cancer memoir to be published in 2014 called *Cleavage to Die For*.

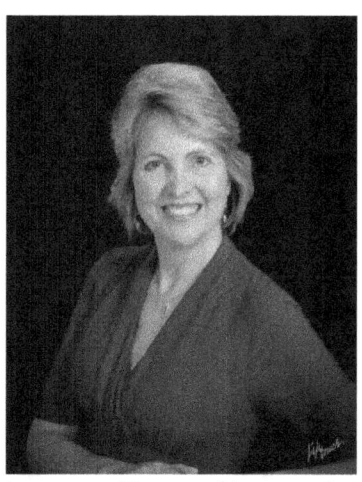

Amy Valentine was a 42-year-old stay-at-home wife and mother of two who had just begun a children's cooking business when she was diagnosed with Stage III bilateral breast cancer. She and her husband Greg were supported by family and friends with special thanks to her wonderful parents, Irv and Jane Smith, who spent countless days caring for the children, taking her to the doctor and providing food and comfort. Amy's caring brother Paul came to all doctor appointments and chemo sessions that Greg couldn't attend. The family's expansive network of friends provided daily care, from bringing meals, visiting her in chemo, stopping by to visit after surgeries, doing laundry, taking care of the children, and many other acts of kindness too numerous to mention. Follow Amy's journey at

www.amyshealth.com

www.ingramcontent.com/pod-product-compliance
Lightning Source LLC
Chambersburg PA
CBHW072254310526
45795CB00012B/1369